NUTRITION & VITAMINS

D1276056

Ann M. Holmes

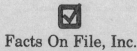

Facts On File, Inc.

Nutrition & Vitamins

Copyright © 1983 by Facts On File, Inc.

The nature of information on nutrition and vitamins is that it is constantly evolving and often subject to interpretation. Therefore, while best efforts have been made to ensure the accuracy and completeness of the information presented, the reader is advised that no claim can be made that all relevant information concerning nutrition and vitamins is included in this book. The reader is reminded that Nutrition & Vitamins *should not be considered a substitute for the professional judgment of a physician or a nutritionist. Facts On File cannot be held responsible for error or for any consequences arising from the use of the information contained herein.*

TABLE OF CONTENTS

Introduction

What is nutrition? Medical dictionaries define it as "the sum of the processes involved in taking in nutriments and assimilating and utilizing them." Sounds simple enough, doesn't it? But today, millions of Americans, as well as millions of people around the world, are obsessed with "good nutrition." The problem is: What constitutes "good nutrition"? Is it grandmother's recipe of "three square meals a day"? Are those who advocate a virtually meatless diet faring better? Do the vegetarians really know something that we don't? Whom should we listen to?

Fortunately, expert advice is available, but sorting it out can be puzzling. To help you understand what good nutrition is all about, we have consulted a number of nutrition experts in order to bring you accurate and up-to-date information. This book discusses all of the major nutrients in detail: proteins, fats and oils, simple and complex carbohydrates, vitamins and minerals. Wherever possible, the recommended daily intake of each is also included. In addition, we have provided pertinent information on fiber and commonly used food additives, as well as several useful charts. We hope you will find this book a truly valuable resource in helping you and your family meet your nutritional needs.

Please remember that information on nutrition is constantly evolving and often subject to a wide variety of interpretations. Therefore, while we have made our best efforts to ensure the accuracy and completeness of the information presented, the reader is reminded that *Nutrition and Vitamins* is not to be considered a substitute for the professional judgment of a physician or a registered nutritionist.

Chapter 1

Nutrition and Health—
The Vital Link

Man is what he eats. Sound trite? Perhaps; but it also has a distinct ring of truth. Everything we eat, from licorice to liquor to that tiny nibble of chocolate cake, passes through the complex maze of the digestive tract. Ultimately, the foods are either utilized by the body's cells and organs, stored for later use or eliminated.

Knowing this, you would think that we would be far more careful about what—and how much—we eat. But we aren't. In fact, when it comes down to day-to-day nutrition, most of us display blasé indifference; for the most part, we blithely ingest all that is placed in front of us, be that three square meals a day or a continental breakfast, coffee break, luncheon, cocktail hour, dinner and a midnight snack.

This blasé attitude is paradoxical, because a recent Harris poll conducted for the Mount Sinai Hospital in Chicago showed that Americans do have a very good idea of what constitutes sound nutritional principles. Nevertheless, we keep right on eating (and eating and eating . . .) virtually anything and everything that comes before us!

Despite our seeming lack of attention to our daily diets, there is ample evidence of the nutrition-health connection—evidence that reveals some alarming trends. For example, even with widespread promotion of numerous products to alleviate "tired" or "iron-poor" blood, iron deficiencies remain this country's most common dietary disorder. In fact, it has been estimated that approximately 5 percent of American women have anemia (a mild iron deficiency).

Other studies also show that, even with our abundant food supply, 1 child in 5 still does not get enough vitamin C each day, and only 1 in 19 takes in an adequate supply of iron. Similarly, studies conducted among Iowa schoolchildren have revealed that those who regularly eat a nutritious breakfast generally do better in school than those who skip out in the morning with perhaps only a doughnut in hand.

2

Although we live in the most "diet-conscious" country in the world, with perhaps more foods to choose from than any other nation, the fact remains that few of us actually associate diet with disease. Nevertheless, our excess consumption of fats (saturated fats, in particular) as well as cholesterol, refined sugar, salt and alcohol has been linked to 6 of the 10 leading causes of death: heart disease, cerebrovascular disease, cancer, diabetes, arteriosclerosis and cirrhosis of the liver. What's more, some experts now believe that a myriad of other medical and behavioral problems—such as fatigue, increased irritability and headache—may also be linked with diet.

As a result of the findings of these and other investigators, many leading health authorities in the United States decided to tackle the problem of nutrition head on. To begin with, they went to the medical schools around the country, only to find that, indeed, very few of them even *offered* courses in nutrition! Thus, medical schools were quickly encouraged to add nutrition courses to their curricula. In addition, a national campaign to overhaul the American "fast-food" diet was begun. The result of these efforts is contained in a government report entitled "U.S. Dietary Goals."

Government-Established Nutrition Goals

Based on studies such as those we have discussed that show the impact of nutrition on health—cardiovascular health, in particular—the U.S. Senate Select Committee on Nutrition and Human Needs established six specific dietary goals for the United States and outlined seven suggestions to help us meet those goals. The goals and their accompanying recommendations are presented below and are illustrated in Figure 1.1.

U.S. Dietary Goals

1. Increase consumption of complex carbohydrates (fruits and vegetables).
2. Decrease consumption of simple carbohydrates.
3. Reduce overall consumption of fats.
4. Specifically, consumption of saturated fats should account for about 10 percent of your total energy intake; that should be balanced with an equal intake of polyunsaturated and monounsaturated fats.
5. Reduce cholesterol consumption to 300 mg per day.
6. Drastically reduce salt consumption to about 3 grams per day.

FIGURE 1.1 *Comparison between current and recommended dietary intake of major nutrients.*

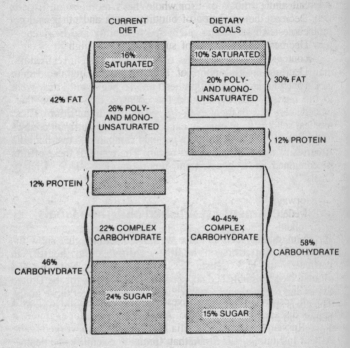

Source: U.S. Senate, Select Committee on Nutrition and Human Needs, "U.S. Dietary Goals," *Dietary Goals for the United States* (Washington, D.C.: U.S. Government Printing Office, December 1977).

Dietary Recommendations

1. Increase consumption of fruits, vegetables and whole grains.
2. Decrease consumption of meat, and increase consumption of poultry and fish.
3. Decrease consumption of foods high in fat and partially substitute polyunsaturated fat for saturated fat.
4. Substitute nonfat milk for whole milk.
5. Decrease consumption of butterfat, eggs and other high-cholesterol sources.
6. Decrease consumption of sugar and foods high in sugar content.
7. Decrease consumption of salt and foods high in salt content.

Lest you think the United States is especially fanatic about health and nutrition, you might be interested to know that governments of the following nine countries have taken similar steps to help their people revise their eating habits and thereby improve their health:

Norway	Australia
Sweden	France
Finland	Germany
United Kingdom	The Netherlands
New Zealand	

What evidence is available to support this? Interestingly enough, researchers began to investigate diet as a possible cause of several diseases many years ago. As early as 1904, for example, a noted Russian researcher, Dr. Ilia Metchnikov, who worked at the Pasteur Institute in Paris, said that "premature senility and death" were for the most part disorders caused by man's "new diet." Essentially, Dr. Metchnikov was referring to the impact of the industrial revolution on man's eating habits.

Shortly after the introduction of machines designed to refine and process foods, many products such as grain and sugar were sent through the mills, where some of the "natural" ingredients such as fiber were removed. As time passed, of course, the processes of refining and food manufacturing became even more sophisticated. Ultimately, virtually every type of food could be refined, processed, preserved, frozen and made reheatable—all in the name of economy and convenience.

A few years later, in agreement with Dr. Metchnikov's hypotheses, Dr. John H. Kellogg, of the Battle Creek, Michigan family whose name is associated with some of today's most popular cereals, argued that diets high in fruits, vegetables, roughage and bran were better for you than eating large quantities of processed foods. Dr. Charles H. Mayo, founder of the world-renowned Mayo Clinic in Minneapolis, concurred. In 1924, in a statement made before the American Medical Association, Dr. Mayo said that Americans

> had been made susceptible to diseases by changes in food that have developed with[in] a few decades; undoubtedly [these changes] have the same relationship to modern life as that which has possibly contributed [to] the increased rate of cancer.

At the time, conventional medicine looked askance at such statements. Many other prominent physicians of the day were in total disagreement with Drs. Kellogg and Mayo, but a massive amount of evidence emerged in the following decades to bear their suspicions out.

Beginning about 1950, epidemiologists and medical researchers began to notice an alarming change in disease and death rates. For no apparent reason, it seemed that the incidence of heart disease, colon cancer, diverticulitis and lung cancer—to name a few—was climbing at a steady rate. Several major studies were undertaken to assess a number of possible causes (diet among them) for this new trend in disease and mortality rates.

Among other things, these studies established the fact that our diets today are in sharp contrast to what our forebears ate. For example, it has been estimated that today every man, woman and child consumes an average of 125 pounds of fat, 188 pounds of meat and 100 pounds of sugar annually. Our consumption of beef has risen sharply, from 55 pounds per person in 1940 to 117 pounds in 1974, an increase of 113 percent. Fat constitutes 42 percent of our total caloric intake—27 percent more fat than our grandparents consumed in 1910. In fact, at the turn of the century, approximately 40 percent of the average daily diet was derived from fresh fruits, vegetables and whole-grain products. Now, only 20 percent of our total calories are consumed from these foods.

In virtually every case the studies mentioned above proved

that the change in man's eating habits could be linked with the changing pattern of disease. Let's take a closer look at some of the specific connections that researchers have established between nutrition and diseases—ranging from relatively minor disorders to known killers.

Sugar-Linked Diseases

Dr. Jean Mayer, currently president of Tufts University Medical Center in Boston, commented in an article in the *Los Angeles Times* in October 1975 that epidemiological studies had linked a high-sugar diet and diabetes. For instance, Yemenite Jewish immigrants to Israel had a low incidence of diabetes—until they consumed a Westernized diet high in sugar for a few years.

Of course, nowhere are the detrimental effects of sugar more obvious than in tooth decay. In the same *Los Angeles Times* article, Dr. Mayer, referring to a government survey, said:

> In nations of the Far East, where sugar intake per person per year ranged (at the time) from 12 to 32 pounds, the national averages for decayed, missing or filled teeth in adults 20 to 24 years old ran from 0.9 to 5. By contrast, in South American nations, where sugar intake was high (44 to 88 pounds per person annually) the averages for decayed, missing or filled teeth in the same age group ran from 8.4 to 12.6. As for the United States today, it has been estimated that 98 percent of American children have some tooth decay; by age 55 about half of the population of this country have no teeth.

Cancer

In June 1979, at the third national meeting on nutritional factors in cancer to be sponsored by the National Cancer Institute and the American Cancer Society, investigators reported that cancers of the stomach, colon, breast, mouth, throat, esophagus, prostate, uterus and ovary have been linked to dietary factors. One medical scientist, Dr. John Weisberger, a member of the American Health Foundation, stated that studies in Japan revealed that frying fish and meats resulted in the formation of chemicals that were structurally related to substances that caused breast and colon cancer in animals. Another investigator, Dr. Ernst Wynder, who is president of the American Health Foundation, said that approximately one-third of all cancers in women and half of the cancers in men were linked to diet.

Dr. Gio Gori then deputy director of the National Cancer Institute, stated in July 1976 before the U.S. Senate's Select Committee on Nutrition and Human Needs:

> There is a strong correlation between dietary fat intake and incidence of breast cancer and colon cancer. As the dietary intake of fat increases, you have an almost linear increase in the incidence of breast and colon cancer....
>
> Colon cancer also has been shown to correlate highly with the consumption of meat, even though it is not clear whether the meat itself or its fat content is the real correlating factor. Mortality rates from colonic cancer are high in the United States, Scotland, and Canada, which are high meat consuming countries; other populations such as Japan and Chile, where meat consumption is low, experience also a low incidence of colon cancer. Seventh Day Adventists and Mormons have a restricted fat and meat intake when compared to other populations living in the same district, and...they suffer considerably less from some forms of cancer, notably breast and colon.

Of course, cancer was a well-recognized disease even 75 years ago, but cancer of the colon and rectum, for example, were considered rare then. Today, statistics from the American Cancer Society show that those cancers virtually tie lung cancer for the highest number of new cases reported annually (excluding common skin cancers).

Cardiovascular Diseases

Dr. Jeremiah Stamler, an internationally recognized authority in epidemiology, nutrition and cardiovascular disease, says we're in the midst of a coronary epidemic. Dr. William Kannel, director of the Framingham Heart Study, calls coronary heart disease "the curse of the 20th century."

Today, it is estimated that approximately one in three men and one in six women in the United States will die from a stroke or heart disease before the age of 60. Yet based on the overwhelming amount of evidence accumulated over the previous two decades or so, a 1971 report prepared by the Department of Agriculture suggested that improving our eating habits could considerably improve our health. In that report, for example, the department estimated that a 25 percent reduction in heart and vasculatory (circulatory) problems could be achieved simply by revising our daily food intake.

Certain studies conducted during World War II are particularly interesting. For example, a noted British nutritionist, Dr. Hugh M. Sinclair, observed that the incidence of heart disease dropped in Rotterdam, Holland during the war, when food rationing was in effect and most people were subjected to egg- and meat-free diets. In postwar Rotterdam, however, the rate of heart disease climbed five times higher than the wartime low and regained the level it had been at prior to the onset of the war.

Similarly, Dr. Ancel Keys, another noted researcher and nutritionist, has spent years studying the role of diet in disease, particularly heart disease. Dr. Keys' studies have revealed, for instance, that Japanese peasants, who eat diets low in saturated fats, have a very low incidence of heart disease. When some of these people moved to Hawaii, however, their dietary intake of saturated fats increased somewhat, as did their incidence of coronary heart disease. But the worst findings appeared when the Japanese moved to the continental United States, where they readily adopted our diet—and developed our incidence of the disease.

The U.S. government has also become increasingly concerned about the incidence of obesity in this country, as well as the association between diets high in animal fats and the incidence of numerous diseases, coronary heart disease in particular. According to most surveys, approximately 20 percent of the adult American population is overweight. In July 1976 Dr. Theodore Cooper, then assistant secretary for health, testified before the Senate Select Committee on Nutrition and Human Needs that these adults were "overweight to a degree that may interfere with optimal health and longevity." The chairman of that committee, Senator George McGovern, said that "the eating patterns of this century represent as critical a public health concern as any now before us."

In general, each country also recommended a reduction in the intake of saturated fat and sugar, as well as advising specific labeling of the fat content in all foods. In fact, as of July 1, 1978, the French Health Ministry began an all-out campaign for a more balanced diet. Like their counterparts in the United States, the French health ministers believe that their countrymen eat too much sugar and fat, and drink too much. According to their findings, the average French citizen also doesn't eat enough whole-grain breads and cereals and all but ignores dry vegetables, such as beans and peas.

What You Can Do

But what steps in particular should you take to achieve these dietary goals? In one word, *modification*—cut down on your intake of saturated or animal fats; reduce your intake of refined and processed foods; and increase your intake of fresh fruits and vegetables, whole-grain breads and cereals, and polyunsaturated fats. The trouble is, you may not be too sure of how to go about doing this without running into a great deal of resistance from your family. Fortunately, drastic changes are not usually needed; most of the dietary modifications that are called for are actually quite simple and basic. Accordingly, here are 20 "tricks" that you can utilize in your family's diet to help you and your family meet the U.S. nutritional goals:

1. Broil or roast meats and fish instead of frying or baking. (Fish can also be poached.)
2. Use margarine instead of butter.
3. Use skim milk instead of whole milk or buttermilk. Give children whole milk, but use skim in recipes.
4. Use bran or sesame-seed toppings instead of bread crumbs. If ambitious, make bread crumbs from whole-grain breads.
5. Season with spices—not salt. Use oregano or thyme instead.
6. Use vinegar or lemon juice with spices instead of heavy oil salad dressings.
7. Serve fresh fruits or yogurt instead of puddings and pies.
8. Use fresh fruits to make your shakes rather than serving sugared sodas.
9. Serve whole-wheat breads instead of white refined-flour breads.
10. Buy tuna packed in water, not oil.
11. Don't overcook vegetables. Vitamins are lost in cooking; the fresher vegetables smell, the more nutritious they are.
12. Don't peel potatoes, cucumbers, apples, pears and so on. The skin is fiber, and the added bulk is good for your digestive tract.
13. Keep nutritious snacks handy. Raisins are advertised as "nature's candy," and other fruits such as pineapples and strawberries would satiate any sweet tooth.
14. Let children snack on sunflower seeds and nuts rather than on sweet cookies.

15. Remove the sugar bowl. If you must use sugar, buy raw sugar.
16. Don't baste meats or other foods with butter; use sesame oil. Dip barbecue brush in it and baste as usual.
17. Use yogurt instead of sour cream in recipes.
18. Before serving chicken, turkey or duck, remove the skin.
19. Trim all excess fat from beef.
20. Buy kosher brands of hot dogs or bologna. These are made from beef, not pork, and are generally less fatty than other brands; they also don't contain additives.

The 20 tricks listed are just a few suggestions. To bring your diet into line with the Senate Select Committee's guidelines, modification is the overall theme. For example, if you tend to eat a lot of canned or processed foods, you should try to incorporate more fresh food items, particularly fruits and vegetables, into your daily diet. Certainly all the ingredients for good nutrition are available to you. For most of us, it simply means paying closer attention to the foods we eat and the beverages we drink; in this country today, there is really no excuse for poor nutritional habits! This book provides you with a considerable amount of information about the essential components of good nutrition. Chapter 12, "Putting It All Together: Now You Be the Nutritionist," tells you how to put this information into a cohesive and nutritionally sound diet plan.

Chapter 2

Proteins

Say "protein" and most Americans automatically think "red meat." In fact, many of us believe, incorrectly, that a "day without protein" is a day quite deficient in the key nutrient. True, protein is an essential nutrient, but it is no more important to adequate nutrition than other nutrients, such as fats and carbohydrates. In addition, it is very difficult for most of us to avoid protein, because the typical diet in the United States today contains approximately 100 grams of protein—62 percent more than a 170-pound person needs for a day! It is far more likely, in fact, that many people are skipping or cutting from their diets essential carbohydrates, based on their belief that carbohydrates are "fattening" but protein can't be skipped.

The Many Roles of Proteins

People seem to be increasingly aware of the importance of protein in their diets, but most of us are less certain of what proteins actually do in the body or how much protein is required.

The word *protein* was coined in 1838 by a Dutch physician and chemist, Jan Mulder. Its derivation is from the Greek *proteios,* meaning "of first importance." Proteins are aptly named because they are present in all living things great and small, plant and animal, and are the "building blocks" of living substance.

As the primary building blocks of the body, proteins are part of every body tissue and fluid. Some organs, like the skin (skin is the largest organ in the body) and its related structures—the hair, fingernails and toenails—are about 98 percent protein. The eyes are protein, as are other major organs of the body, such as the heart, liver and kidneys. Cell walls throughout the body are made up of protein, and the bulk of cell contents is protein. Proteins are also the major components of muscle tissue, and most of the body fluids and secretions are proteins. This includes pancreatic secretion and insulin as well as various secretions of the thyroid gland and the pituitary. Digestive and other enzymes are proteins; so are antibodies. In addition, many of the blood constituents are proteins—the hemoglobin of the red blood cells, which transports oxygen to cells throughout the body; proteins that transport nutrients in the bloodstream; and albumin, which aids in maintaining the proper balance between acidity and alkalinity (referred to as pH) as well as fluid balance. Proteins also help to form hormones, which have such diverse functions as regulating growth, sexual maturation, reproductive cycles, pregnancy and lactation, plus a host of other functions. Even the genes that determine the form and fate of future generations are proteins— and these are just some of the multiple roles of proteins.

Although proteins are "building blocks," they may also be used to produce energy when they are in excess or when adequate amounts of carbohydrates are not available. We will discuss this use of proteins later.

In summary, proteins serve these multiple functions:

- To develop and repair tissues
- To transport oxygen and nutrients
- To manufacture enzymes and hormones
- To aid in formation of blood clots
- To maintain normal pH and fluid balance
- To provide needed nitrogen and carbon
  - Nitrogen for manufacture of nitrogenous compounds
  - Carbon as central structure for glucose (when necessary) and certain nonessential amino acids synthesized by the body
- To provide energy under certain circumstances

Amino Acids

Although each plant and animal species contains a number of its own unique proteins, all proteins have basic similarities. Proteins are complex chemical compounds with thousands of atoms linked in various ways so that each type of protein molecule has its own pattern. Like fats and carbohydrates, proteins contain carbon, hydrogen and oxygen; but unlike fats and carbohydrates, they also contain nitrogen, whose importance we will discuss later.

The basic unit of all proteins is the amino acid. When one considers the vast numbers of proteins found in nature, it is remarkable that there are only 20 or so amino acids. Yet the variety of proteins is made possible by the different lengths of the amino acid chains, their varied combinations and the manner in which they are joined. Perhaps even more remarkable is the fact that all proteins are composed of water, air, soil and sunlight converted by plants and certain protozoa into living substance.

The Essential Amino Acids

Approximately 20 (from 18 to 22) amino acids are said to be commonly found in foods, but the only ones called "essential" are those that the body cannot make itself from the nitrogenous portions of ingested proteins (See Table 2.1). This means that these amino acids must be *preformed* (already present in this form) in foods we eat.

Nine amino acids are classified as "essential." These are the following:

TABLE 2.1
AMINO ACIDS

Essential	Isoleucine
	Leucine
	Lysine
	Methionine
	Phenylalanine
	Threonine
	Tryptophan
	Valine
Essential for Infants	Histidine
Nonessential	Glycine
	Glutamic acid
	Arginine
	Aspartic acid
	Proline
	Alanine
	Serine
	Tyrosine
	Cysteine
	Asparagine
	Glutamine
	Hydroxyproline
	Citrulline

Although histidine has long been thought important only for infants, recent studies have suggested that some histidine may be required for adults. Arginine, sometimes cited as being essential for children, is not recognized as such by the National Academy of Sciences. Tyrosine and cystine, although considered "nonessential," are to some degree able to be interconverted with methionine and phenylalanine, respectively, thereby lowering the requirements of these amino acids.

The changing data are reflective of continuing research in the field, where, as in all dynamic fields, knowledge is continually updated and revised.

Proteins are not usable as complete molecules. The body must break them down into amino acids, which can be absorbed into the bloodstream. Once in the bloodstream, those amino acids needed for growth and repair are selected according to the needs of the individual cells and tissues. Proteins uniquely suited to the body are then constructed from these amino acids.

When the selection is not exactly according to the body's needs, the body can construct its own amino acids by a process called "transamination." In this process, the liver "steals" an amino group from one amino acid and the acid group from another amino acid and makes the desired amino acid. But one amino acid cannot substitute for another, nor can the body construct necessary proteins unless the requisite amino acids or their components are available from dietary intake.

About 80 percent of an individual's daily protein requirement is used to synthesize amino acids the body can make itself. The remaining 20 percent of the daily requirement is for essential amino acids. The body's protein needs, then, are divided into two parts:

1. The need for dietary nitrogen to enable the body to make its own proteins and amino acids.
2. The need for preformed "essential" amino acids.

Obviously, foods supplying the "essential" amino acids could be consumed in quantities sufficient to supply all dietary protein needs, but this would be very costly and wasteful. The nitrogen would simply be stripped from the protein molecule and the remainder burned for energy, stored as fat or discarded.

Complete and Incomplete Proteins

In terms of supplying essential amino acids, all proteins are not equal. This idea is expressed in terms of "complete" versus "incomplete" proteins. Complete proteins supply required amounts of *all* of the essential amino acids, whereas incomplete proteins do not. Most, although not *all*, of the complete proteins are from animal sources—meat, fish, eggs, dairy products—while most of the incomplete proteins are from plant sources, such as leafy green and yellow vegetables. Only refined carbohydrates such as sugars and cornstarch and refined fats like butter and oils are completely devoid of protein. In order to receive complete protein, two or more incomplete proteins must be consumed together—for example, beans and rice—or a small amount of a complete protein such as eggs can be added to an incomplete protein.

Since proteins are in almost all the foods we eat, it is nearly impossible to avoid having ample protein in the diet—at least in the typical diet of someone in the United States. But what about complete proteins for vegetarians? What about the relatively expensive sources of complete proteins for those with slim pocketbooks?

Fortunately for the less affluent—and that includes most of the world's population—the body's wisdom extends to the acceptance of two or more incomplete proteins in place of more expensive complete proteins. As mentioned, the body breaks down all proteins into their amino acids. Once in the bloodstream, there is no way to tell whether the amino acid had an originally prestigious source or a relatively humble one. Nor does the body care. Identical amino acids are equal in terms of the body's needs.

Many countries have solved the problem of adequate nutrition with little or no reliance on animal sources. Table 2.2 lists some familiar combinations of foods that meet these criteria. It should be mentioned that although milk is an honored protein source in the United States, in many parts of Europe (especially the Scandinavian countries and the Lowlands), and among certain African tribes such as the Masai, it is by no means a habitual drink throughout most of the world. It has been somewhat facetiously remarked that "cow's milk is only good for baby cows," and to some degree this is true. Many Oriental people, some Mediterranean people and most African blacks are unable to digest cow's milk because they lack an enzyme called lactase. This enzyme is apparently present in these populations during the years when they would normally be expected to be drinking their own mother's milk. In populations continuing to drink milk into adulthood, the enzyme persists. One occasionally sees articles concerning the so-called lactase deficiency in various populations, but perhaps the persistence of lactase may be the abnormality, not vice versa.

TABLE 2.2

COMMON COMBINATIONS OF FOODS PROVIDING COMPLETE PROTEINS IN REQUIRED AMOUNTS

Rice and beans	— Latin America
Rice and peas	— the Caribbean
Wheat and peas, beans or lentils	— India
Wheat bread and cheeses	— Western and Middle Eastern countries
Pasta and beans	— Mediterranean countries
Rice and soy products	— Oriental countries
Corn and beans	— North America (American Indians and other North Americans)
Cereal and milk	— North America

Nonetheless, milk serves an important function in the American diet, not only as a protein source but as a source of calcium and vitamin D.

Vegetarianism and Protein Needs

Vegetarians of all kinds have used the technique of combining various foods to make complete, interesting and nutritious diets. There are some caveats, however, for those who prefer, for one reason or another, to avoid animal sources of protein. Some vegetarians, for example, simply avoid meats, fish and poultry, retaining both eggs and dairy products in their diet. These vegetarians are called ovolactovegetarians, and their proteins closely resemble those of persons eating a regular diet. Vegans, on the other hand, do not include eggs, milk or any dairy products in their diet. These people may have some difficulties not only in regard to getting enough protein from their diet, but also in getting enough of vitamins D and B_{12}. The ways to meet these vitamin needs, so vital in pregnant women, growing children and teenagers, are discussed in the chapter on vitamins.

If you avoid meats, and especially if you are a vegan, some planning is needed to make certain that essential proteins are included without the need for excessive caloric intake or bulk. A sample menu is shown here for a typical day. In this case, the only changes necessary for vegans would be to substitute soy milk or fruit juice for the milk at breakfast.

BREAKFAST
Oatmeal with milk and fruit
Orange juice
2 slices of whole wheat toast with apple butter

LUNCH
Peanut butter and jam sandwich on whole wheat bread
Vegetable-barley soup

DINNER
Pasta with broccoli, mushrooms and pignolis
Large salad with dressing

The menu shown suits the nutritional needs of a healthy 170-pound male who requires 2,650 calories daily as maintenance and whose protein requirement (recommended dietary allowance) is for 61.6 grams. Sources of concentrated proteins for many vegetarians and those desiring good, relatively low-cost protein sources are listed here:

Legumes—soybeans, lentils, garbanzos, peas, pinto beans, etc.

Cheeses—most cheeses, including Swiss, cheddar, parmesan, cottage cheese and ricotta

Other foods—eggs, wheat germ, wheat bran

Less common foods—soy grits or flour, torula or brewer's yeast, gluten flour, tofu (bean curd)

Although it is not recommended, there is some evidence that the body is capable of going for a comparatively long time on a relatively protein-deficient diet, without suffering adverse effects. One study conducted about 60 years ago showed that a group of men were capable of maintaining themselves quite well on wheat bread alone. Other studies have been done with similar results, giving subjects only potatoes. Perhaps the reason for these findings lies in the fact that the human intestine itself can serve as a source of high-quality protein. According to studies, the sloughed-off lining plus the protein of the intestinal enzymes can supply up to 90 grams of high-quality protein daily.

Animal Versus Non-Animal Proteins

Are animal-derived proteins superior to those derived from non-animal sources? Are non-animal protein sources superior? Does it matter? Not surprisingly, both views are supported by very vocal groups, each with some persuasive and valid arguments. Let's take a look at the pros and cons.

Economy

There is absolutely no doubt that in most areas of the world animal-derived protein is far more costly. Eskimos and tribes living at the polar extremities might well take issue with this stance, but admittedly, their situation is unique. There is also a persuasive argument that since all protein is derived in the long run from plant sources, it is cheaper to eat plants to start with than to feed the plants to animals and then eat the animals. Then there is the moral question of whether this expensive sequence should be maintained for a minority of the Earth's population when hunger is such a widespread global phenomenon. Unfortunately, worldwide hunger cannot be alleviated by individual decisions to eat or not eat particular foods. Larger issues are at stake. One can only hope that those in whose power it is to make such decisions and plans will opt for realistic arrangements that will truly benefit the starving peoples of the world.

Better Grade of Protein

It must be conceded that, with one exception (gelatin), the animal-derived proteins are complete proteins, thereby eliminating the problem of having to construct combinations of incomplete proteins. The task is even more difficult for vegetarians who do not eat either eggs or dairy products.

Quantity Needed

Vegetarians need to consume more calories to supply their protein needs than meat eaters do. For example, you would have to drink a quart of milk to receive the same amount of protein as four ounces of meat. But curiously, vegetarians are usually thinner than meat eaters because the bulk found in vegetables fills them up quickly. They therefore tend to eat less. Because so much of their daily food intake must be used to receive the needed amount of proteins, they must be extremely careful to balance their diets so that they receive all the nutrients their bodies need.

Similarity to Human Protein

Obviously, animal proteins are more similar to human proteins than plant proteins; however, since all proteins must be broken down to their amino acids before the body can use them, it is questionable whether or not this is of importance.

Digestibility

Digestibility depends on which proteins are being discussed. The fact is that nutritionists divide proteins into three categories, depending on complexity. Both animal and plant proteins appear in each of the three groups. *Simple proteins* (for example, albumin, globulins and wheat glutens) when broken down yield only amino acids. *Compound proteins* contain amino acids plus fats, carbohydrates, etc. *Derived proteins* are those produced by the breakdown of compound proteins. The relative complexity or simplicity of these proteins is unrelated to whether or not the proteins are complete. For example, zein (found in corn) is an incomplete protein, while albumin (found in eggs) is a complete protein that is often regarded as the ideal protein food.

A significant portion of plant proteins may be indigestible and lost in the feces; the body best absorbs animal proteins, but many of these may be accompanied by large amounts of saturated fats, which may not only be difficult to digest but may lead to another set of problems (see Chapter 3). Lean meats are obviously easier to digest.

Excessive Weight Gain

Advocates of plant protein point out that animal protein frequently contains large amounts of fat. However, those favoring animal sources of protein indicate that people *need* fat (at least in moderation) and that it is easier to stay slim or become slim on a protein-rich diet than on one that requires concomitant ingestion of large amounts of carbohydrates.

Obviously, selection of protein sources and moderation in amounts of food eaten are key elements in any diet. Certainly there is a danger in overeating of animal proteins to the point where nutrients required from plant sources will not be obtained— there won't be any *room* to eat more. People who stuff themselves with high-bulk vegetables, on the other hand, may shortchange themselves on proteins.

Efficiency

Nutritionists rate the quality (nutritive value) of a protein on both digestibility and biological value (the amino acid composition), the so-called NPU (net protein utilization). This number is then compared with protein similar to egg white, which offers all of the essential amino acids in a simple and readily digested form. The higher the NPU, the closer to this ideal protein. Obviously, animal proteins generally possess higher NPU numbers. It is also obvious that considering NPU alone is not the full story. Good nutrition demands more than efficient sources of protein. By combining foods, one can obtain high-quality protein from readily available and economical sources that individually might have relatively low NPU numbers.

Protein Needs in the Normal, Healthy Adult

The human body has been compared to a city, which, once built, requires constant repair and rebuilding. After all, cells cannot live forever, and with the exception of certain nerve cells that do not regenerate, body cells are in a constant state of turnover. Skin cells, for example, are continually being born in the lower layer of the skin and migrating to upper layers, where as dead cells they are worn away and washed away, only to be replaced with those immediately beneath them. Red blood cells live out their brief life span (approximately four months) and then must be replaced by new carriers of oxygen. White blood cells live their usually short and hard lives fighting bacteria and other invaders; some explode, triggering the inflammatory process, which entraps the hapless invader, while others engulf and swallow all foreign material and debris and die in the process. Whenever possible, the body efficiently recycles the protein, but inevitably, some is lost. There is no way for the body to recapture and recycle the protein from hair. Once it has grown out, it is no longer living material. Like nail parings and dead skin, hair is a "dead loss." Body secretions and fluids such as menstrual flow, semen and mucous secretions from various body openings as well as proteins in the urine and feces are also lost to recycling.

Protein Requirements

Although the needs of the average adult for protein to repair tissues and replace those that are worn out are obviously not as great as for individuals who are building new tissues, the need is continuous. Differences in daily protein requirements of various groups are reflected in the recommended daily allowances (RDAs), as set forth by the Food and Nutrition Board of the National Academy of Sciences. Although admittedly incomplete, these values are based on nutritional information applicable to many healthy people and are not intended to represent therapeutic recommendations in any case. There has been some criticism that the recommended levels are only life-sustaining and not health-sustaining and certainly not sufficient to prevent degenerative disease, at least in terms of vitamin and mineral recommendations. Then again, some consider the recommended protein allowances too high, while others consider them too low. Perhaps it would be wise to regard RDAs as guidelines only, not as the last word on the subject. One recent text for physicians and other medical professionals offered the following list of reasons for regarding the RDAs as being of limited value:

- Many of the values are based on short-term studies of blood or tissue levels of a substance or short-term balance studies (e.g., nitrogen balance to evaluate protein intake) or are based on minimal amounts of the substance required to prevent frank symptoms of deficiency.
- Many studies are done on young, healthy men, and from these values approximations have been made as to the needs of special groups such as women, growing children and the elderly.
- Interactions between certain nutrients and food constituents that might affect the availability of some nutrients are not taken into consideration.
- Only about one-third of the essential nutrients have any RDAs.
- Individual differences in physical activity, physiologic state or therapeutic needs are not considered.

The latest RDAs for protein are listed in Table 2.3. For infants, the RDAs are listed in grams of protein for each kilogram of body weight per day, and for other groups as grams per day. For pregnant and lactating women, figures listed recommend at least that amount, with the plus indicating more than the minimum figure.

So much for RDAs. What are USRDAs? These are values based on the RDAs and meant as standards for nutritional labeling of commercially sold foods. A glance at the packaging of various foods displayed in any market will show a nutritional value listing that indicates that they provide a certain percentage of the protein, vitamins, minerals, etc., determined to be required in the daily diet. Obviously, since people's requirements are not all alike, neither can the percentages of their requirements be alike. The Food and Drug Administration has therefore arbitrarily determined the average need to be that of the highest level of requirement of an adult male. In this way, it is hoped that the minimum needs of most will be met, even allowing for special stresses that can alter requirements. Imperfect though this may be, at least manufacturers must indicate the "known quantities" of those nutrients for which RDAs have been established.

TABLE 2.3
RECOMMENDED DIETARY ALLOWANCES FOR PROTEIN*

	Age (years)	Weight (kg)	Weight (lb)	Height (cm)	Height (in)	Protein (g)
Infants	0.0 – 0.5	6	13	60	24	kg × 2.2
	0.5 – 1.0	9	20	71	28	kg × 2.0
Children	1 – 3	13	29	90	35	23
	4 – 6	20	44	112	44	30
	7 – 10	28	62	132	52	34
Males	11 – 14	45	99	157	62	45
	15 – 18	66	145	176	69	56
	19 – 22	70	154	177	70	56
	23 – 50	70	154	178	70	56
	51 +	70	154	178	70	56
Females	11 – 14	46	101	157	62	46
	15 – 18	55	120	163	64	46
	19 – 22	55	120	163	64	44
	23 – 50	55	120	163	64	44
	51 +	55	120	163	64	44
Pregnant						+ 30
Lactating						+ 20

*The allowances are intended to provide for individual variations among most normal persons as they live in the United States under usual environmental stresses. Diets should be based on a variety of common foods in order to provide other nutrients for which human requirements have been less well defined.

SOURCE: National Academy of Sciences, Committee on Dietary Allowances, Food and Nutrition Board, *Recommended Dietary Allowances,* 9th revised ed. (Washington, D.C., 1980).

What About Minimum Daily Requirements (MDRs)?

One seldom sees the MDR designation today. At one time the minimum daily requirements, established by the Food and Drug Administration, served the same purpose as the USRDAs do now. Although MDRs are obsolete standards, they may occasionally be seen on some cereal labels.

Timing Protein Intake

At one time, people thought that in order for the body to utilize the essential amino acids properly, they all had to be present in foods eaten at the same time. This theory was based on experiments with rats, in which it was shown that if complementary amino acids were given hours apart, the infant rats had impaired growth. However, more recent studies and reexamination of previous findings have caused a change in opinion. First of all, infant rats being fed purified amino acids cannot be compared with humans eating food. Second, the more immediate growth needs of a rapidly growing animal with a short life span cannot be compared with usual human dietary needs. It is now thought that as long as all of the essential amino acids are consumed daily, they need not be eaten at the same meal. Explanations are offered that every cell has amino acids in its interior that can be called upon to supply temporary needs for essential amino acids, and then later replaced. Additionally, the aforementioned ability of intestinal mucosa to supply essential amino acids may help to make up for the deficit if there is a lag in consumption.

A wide selection of foods and intelligent moderation in selecting them should permit an adequate intake of all nutrients, whether one opts for animal or plant-sourced proteins or a combination.

Time of Increased Protein Requirements

Additional proteins are needed during periods of rapid growth, during times of special physiologic stress (during strenuous exercise, for example) and when there are greater than usual repair and maintenance requirements (for instance, during an illness).

The normal, healthy adult in the United States consumes sufficient protein to meet usual needs and eliminates a corresponding amount of nitrogen. When intake equals output, the body is considered in nitrogen equilibrium, which is the normal state. A positive nitrogen balance exists when more protein is taken in than nitrogen is eliminated. Positive nitrogen balance is necessary during pregnancy because added proteins must be retained to meet both fetal and maternal needs. It is imperative that these needs be filled because fetal needs will be met first, even to the extent of drawing from maternal supplies to the detriment of the mother.

Growing children and teen-agers should also be in positive nitrogen balance because of their increased growth needs. While growth may be more obvious in early childhood and the protein needs clearly evident, increasing protein requirements persist until adulthood. Much of the new growth in older children may be in changes due to sexual maturation rather than structural growth.

During periods of conditioning, athletes are also in positive nitrogen balance because additional muscle mass is being produced. As training continues and optimal conditioning renders further muscle growth unnecessary, the nitrogen balance gradually returns to a state of equilibrium.

Lactating women, although they lose as much nitrogen daily as they take in, appear to be in positive balance because they are creating high-quality protein breast milk, which is consumed daily by the nursing infant.

A negative nitrogen balance is generally a pathologic state and can be due to a number of causes, such as illness, injury or starvation. As the condition is remedied, the individuals are in a temporary state of positive nitrogen balance until the situation is reversed and equilibrium restored.

Prolonged negative nitrogen balance is incompatible with life; the body consumes itself in a frantic effort to keep pace with the rapidly increasing need for proteins. Gross malnutrition, severe burns, debilitating illnesses and extensive trauma and blood loss are examples of such life-threatening conditions.

Otherwise healthy individuals who are "crash" dieting or fasting for one reason or another will be in temporary negative nitrogen balance. The longer such situations continue, the more serious are the possible consequences. Recently, in response to the fad for "fasting" diets, many people placed themselves on "starvation" diets and bought over-the-counter forms of "protein supplements" to take during the day; little, if any, food was consumed. A number of deaths were subsequently attributed to this type of fasting-supplement diet, and ultimately, many of these protein-supplement products were removed from the market.

Although "fasting" can be used as a means of weight loss, strict monitoring by a physician is necessary, and even then, these diets are only indicated for the grossly obese individual. In some cases, physicians recommend hospitalization, so they can monitor the individual closely; in other cases, the patient may simply be asked to return to the physician for weekly or biweekly checkups.

Clearly, both negative and positive nitrogen balance call for increased protein intake, in the former case to repair and rebuild and in the latter for new growth.

High-Protein Diets

Although there is some disagreement as to the exact amount of protein required daily, it is conceded that pregnant women, nursing mothers, growing children and persons recovering from illnesses require additional dietary proteins. Men also require more protein than women. There is also some disagreement about whether persons who do hard physical labor require more protein than others. Based on nitrogen loss (which some regard as a less than satisfactory way to measure protein consumption and protein needs), there would appear to be little need for such extra proteins. However, as shown in Table 2.4, laborers in many countries are regarded as needing substantial extra quantities of protein. Perhaps considering the laborer as one would consider an athlete is a way of approaching the problem. But there is no unanimity here, either. As previously mentioned, during the training period there is an increased need for proteins as increased muscle mass is accumulated with exercise. However, protein overload past these needs is of doubtful value and may even be harmful. A number of undesirable effects of protein overload have been documented:

- *Concomitant low carbohydrates,* leading to muscle breakdown and release of myoglobin into the bloodstream, resulting in loss of storage protein for the muscles.
- *Ketosis* (an abnormally elevated concentration of ketone [acetone] bodies in body tissues and fluids) *and dehydration* due to low carbohydrate intake and increased urination.
- *Iron loss* because myoglobin contains iron.
- *Calcium loss*
- *Enlarged liver* because the liver must work harder to "deaminate" (remove) the excessive amounts of amino acids.
- *Enlarged kidneys* because of the extra work required to clear large amounts of urea from the blood. The large quantities of urea are formed in converting the ammonia (a toxic substance) formed during deamination to a substance

TABLE 2:4
PROTEIN NEEDS FOR LABORERS

Country	Recommended Grams of Protein Daily
Sweden	189
Russia	132
Germany	145
Italy	115
France	135
England	151
United States—men (no specific recommendation for type of work)	56
—women (no work specification)	55

(urea) capable of being carried away from the body by the kidneys. (An inflammation of the kidneys has been noted in some animals with a high-protein diet.) It should be mentioned that gout can result with high urea levels in some people in whom urea is converted to uric acid.

* *Low dietary fiber* is characteristic of high-protein diets, and dietary fiber appears to play an important role in digestion and healthy intestines.

* *Possible excessive cell turnover.* It has been suggested that very high amino acid levels in the blood may increase cell protein turnover and that this heightened metabolic rate causes cells to age faster.

Adequate quantities of hydrochloric acid (HCl) in the stomach are required to digest any protein. Most people are more aware of the problems of excessive hydrochloric acid as graphically portrayed on television. The problem is that the feeling of a "lump in the stomach" may be due to either too much or not enough hydrochloric acid. Certain illnesses, stress and increased age can cause a lack of hydrochloric acid, although some babies also have the problem. In addition, vitamin and/or mineral deficiencies can cause a lack of HCl. Some trial-and-error methods can be used to see whether one's problem is due to an excess or a lack of stomach acid.

Protein Supplements—Who Needs Them?

It seems difficult to justify the use of protein supplements for those in good health and with no special reason to need added proteins. The fallacy of needing extra proteins for "energy" is quite transparent. Carbohydrates are the most efficient source of energy, and even complex carbohydrates are metabolized more rapidly than proteins. So much for "fast energy" from proteins. Protein supplements can be very important, however, for those recovering from illness and those undergoing stress that depletes the body's resources. Children who fail to thrive are often given supplementation in liquid form, and high-protein liquid diets liberally laced with other important nutrients may be considered preferable to intravenous feedings for those unable to eat. But the much-touted "special energy" foods and beverages that athletes and other active people supposedly require have more promotion than fact behind their claims.

Symptoms of Protein Deficiency

Severe protein deficiency usually accompanies general severe malnutrition. Certainly the pictures of famine-ravaged and war-torn countries and huge-eyed, swollen-bellied children are familiar to everyone, though few Americans have firsthand experience with starvation. Middle-class Americans may be more familiar with the signs of relative starvation of some of the very fashionably thin models, ballet stars and troubled teen-agers. Malnutrition of a different kind can be seen more readily in junk-food addicts, many of whom are overweight, pasty-skinned, low in energy with little resistance to infection. Poorly fed infants and children are a familiar sight in every hospital and clinic—many of these children being described simply as "failing to thrive." Such a nonspecific classification may include many with protein deficiency. In a more radical and visible form, this disease is called "kwashiorkor" and is commonly seen in many parts of the world where the older child becomes ill when the mother has another baby to breast-feed. Since milk was the child's chief or only protein source, and it becomes unavailable, it is not long before symptoms become apparent. "Kwashiorkor" is specific protein deficiency, as opposed to "marasmus," which occurs with multi-nutrient deprivation seen in starvation.

Prolonged deprivation, not surprisingly, affects all parts of the body. In young children, brain development can be retarded, leading to permanent mental retardation even if adequate nutrition is restored. Behavioral difficulties and nervous instability are common. Protein-deficient people tend to be irritable, listless and weak, with easy fatigability. They are anemic and show signs of muscle wasting, which can be disguised somewhat by the bloated appearance due to water retention. Circulation is poor; blood pressure is abnormally low; wound healing is prolonged; and constipation is a common complaint. Kidney and liver complications are common, as is peptic ulcer. Understandably, there is little resistance to infection. Vision is poor, and many suffer from the symptoms of low blood sugar.

Obviously, not all people will experience all of these symptoms, but early signs of some of these disorders can be seen in unwary dieters, young people with "anorexia nervosa"—a disease in which extremely thin individuals perceive themselves as fat and consequently refuse to eat—people who eat refined starches and sugars to the exclusion of more nutritious foods, and uninformed vegetarians. Symptoms may also be common in persons with chronic wasting illnesses. In the absence of debilitating illness or psychological disturbances necessitating strict medical supervision, most people can prevent or correct protein deficiency, perhaps with some guidance from a doctor or a registered dietitian. In most instances, misguided efforts to lose weight are the initial cause of insufficient nutrition in otherwise normal people.

The Bottom Line on Proteins

Proteins are vital nutrients for any balanced diet. As we have heard since childhood, they are the building blocks of the body, the components of living substances. For a large number of Americans a meal is not complete without protein, particularly animal protein. We look upon meat as a major component of our diet, necessary for vitality and for maintaining or achieving a slim figure. But as we have seen, we can get the vital amino acids we must have from a wide variety of foods. Whole grains, vegetables and legumes, in the right proportions, can give us the complete proteins we need without the drawbacks that animal proteins have with their often high amounts of fat. And while we may not want to dismiss meat from our diet, we would all do well to diversify our sources of protein. We would thereby add variety to our diet—and probably save money.

Chapter 3

Fats and Cholesterol

One of the most controversial areas of nutrition is the one that deals with fats and cholesterol and their effects on human health. There are differing views and conflicting evidence, and several serious questions have been raised: Are fats good for us? Or the opposite? Are saturated fats harmful? And what about cholesterol? Given our bodies' production of cholesterol, does it matter how much we consume in our diet? Most people have heard that a high intake of saturated fats and cholesterol causes heart disease. How warranted are such charges? Do fats and cholesterol play a role in the causation of cancer?

This chapter will attempt to answer these questions. The answers will, of necessity, be tentative, but enough is known to allow some recommendations on the place of fats and cholesterol in a healthful diet. Before talking about health, though, we should examine what fats and cholesterol are and how they function in the body.

Fats and cholesterol belong to a diverse group of organic compounds known as lipids. These compounds are distinguished by the fact that they are soluble not in water but in certain organic solvents, such as ether, benzene and ethanol. This affects their digestion and their transport in the body, topics that will be discussed later in the chapter.

Fats: What They Are and Why They Are Important

Fats, like carbohydrates, contain carbon, hydrogen and oxygen atoms. (Protein contains these three elements plus nitrogen.) The proportions of carbon, hydrogen and oxygen differ in fats and carbohydrates: fats contain less oxygen and more carbon and hydrogen than do carbohydrates. This means that fats burn more completely. A gram of carbohydrate (or protein) yields about four calories; a gram of fat yields nine calories.

To put this another way, fats are the most concentrated sources of dietary energy. Because of this fact, it is easy to overindulge, and by and large, this is precisely what we do. Americans obtain more than 40 percent of their calories from fats. Opinions vary on what share fats should have in our diet, but numerous studies have indicated that our present intake is too high and that we have nothing to lose by lowering it.

One simple reason we overindulge in fats is because they make most food taste better; many of the pleasing flavors and smells of food come from fats. Fats are often responsible for our feeling "full," sometimes unpleasantly so, long after eating certain foods. The reason is because fats take longer to digest than either carbohydrates or protein. (Chinese food has little fat compared with other cuisines; this is why people sometimes complain of feeling hungry not long after eating a Chinese meal.)

Dietary and Body Fats

We encounter fats in the foods we eat and, even more intimately, in ourselves. "Dietary fats" is the term used for the former and "body fats" designates the latter.

Fat in meat and poultry is readily recognizable, and some other foods, such as butter, lard and oils, are all fat. (Fats that are in a liquid state at 20 degrees centigrade are usually termed oils.) However, not all dietary fats are so apparent; nuts and avocados, for example, are very high in fat content. Table 3.1 compares the fat content of different foods.

Dietary fats are broken down in the digestive process and reassembled for various purposes; they don't necessarily make a beeline for the paunch or hips. Body fat is located in different places in the body: the liver, around various organs, and—all too often—in unwanted bulges and rolls. It can be thought of as a form of stored energy; if we eat more calories than we burn off on a day-to-day basis, we "get" fat. There is no need to eat a lot of fat in order to get fat, however: excess calories in whatever form are converted to fat.

What Fat Does for Us

Contemporary fashion makes few allowances for fat. Moreover, fat is frequently blamed as a cause of health problems. Nevertheless, it performs some essential functions in the body.

First, stored energy—fat—is something we all need. We don't eat constantly, so we must have a reserve that can be called upon when required; even the thinnest people have some body fat. In addition, body fat provides a protective, cushioning layer around important organs: the heart, liver, kidneys and intestine. Without such protection, all these organs would be vulnerable to frequent injury.

The fat that lies just under the skin, called subcutaneous fat, also serves as insulation against extremes of heat and cold. As a person grows older, the layers of subcutaneous fat generally grow thinner, making the bony structures of the hands, face, neck and feet more prominent. Aging also causes a person's fat to become less evenly distributed—this is part of the reason why many older people are acutely sensitive to the cold.

Body fats are responsible for attractive, lively hair and smooth skin. Women who do not have adequate body fat can suffer a disruption of their reproductive cycles and hormone balance.

From the viewpoint of nutrition, dietary fats perform two key functions:

- They enable the body to absorb and utilize the vitamins A, D, E and K, which are fat-soluble.
- They provide linoleic acid, which is known as the essential fatty acid. (Fatty acids are a component of fats, as will be explained shortly.)

Linoleic acid is a component of the fats found in corn oil and some other vegetable oils. Two other fatty acids—arachidic acid and linolenic acid—are described by some writers as essential, but this is not strictly true, since the body can manufacture both if it is supplied with enough linoleic acid. Linoleic, arachidic and linolenic acid play an important part in the manufacture of both phospholipids, which help to form cell membranes, and prostaglandins. While prostaglandins are relatively new to medical science, they appear to be involved in the regulation of blood pressure; the "stickiness" of blood platelets, which are essential to the blood-clotting process; and the onset of labor. Although linoleic acid is vital to the body's functioning, only a small quantity is required. It should supply 1 percent to 2 percent of a person's daily calories, which can be obtained from a tablespoon of corn oil, soybean oil or certain other vegetable oils.

Saturated and Unsaturated Fats

Most of the criticism of fats on health grounds is directed against a particular group: the saturated fats, which are distinguished from unsaturated fats by their chemical structure. Let's look at what the difference is.

Fat molecules, both saturated and unsaturated, have two components: glycerol and fatty acids. Glycerol, also known as glycerine, is a greasy alcohol; it is, as might be guessed, an ingredient of nitroglycerin and is used in making many other substances as well. Fatty acids belong to a major class of organic compounds known as carboxylic acids.

If the glycerol part is joined to only one fatty acid, the resultant molecule is called a monoglyceride. A fat molecule with two fatty acids is termed a diglyceride, and one with three fatty acids is called a triglyceride. Triglycerides, which are by far the most important, account for about 95 percent of both the animal and vegetable fats in our diet.

It is the fatty acid part of the molecule that is either saturated or unsaturated. For our purposes, it is sufficient to think of a fatty acid as a chain of carbon atoms with hydrogen atoms attached. Each carbon atom can form bonds with four other atoms; alternatively, it can form links with three other atoms, one of the links being a double bond.

The more double bonds there are, the fewer hydrogen atoms. (The trade-off is always between hydrogen atoms and double bonds; dropping a carbon atom would mean a break in the chain that makes up the fatty acid.) A *saturated* fat is simply one in which the fatty acids have no double bonds—that is, one in which there are as many hydrogen atoms as possible. (The fat is "saturated" with hydrogen.) An unsaturated fat has one or more double bonds. Fatty acids with one double bond are termed *monounsaturated;* those with two or more are called *polyunsaturated.*

Figure 3.1 shows both a saturated and a polyunsaturated string of carbon atoms. (Single bonds are shown as a dash; double bonds as an equal sign.)

With some important exceptions, animal fats tend to have a high proportion of saturated fats, while vegetables generally have monounsaturated or polyunsaturated fats.

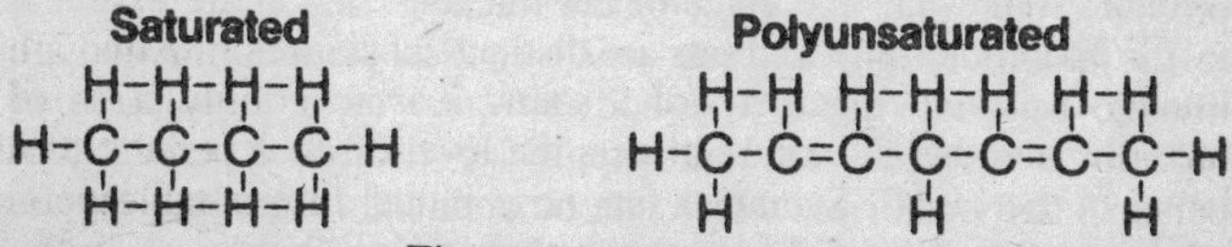

Saturated

```
    H--H--H--H
H--C--C--C--C--H
    H--H--H--H
```

Polyunsaturated

```
    H--H  H--H--H  H--H
H--C--C=C--C--C=C--C--H
    H         H        H
```

Figure 3.1 *Fatty Acids*

Hydrogenation

The degree of saturation affects how solid a fat is at room temperature. At this temperature, foods with a high proportion of saturated fats, such as butter, are fairly firm; those composed mainly of polyunsaturated fats—corn oil, for example—are liquid.

We are accustomed to thinking of corn oil as a liquid, but in some other foods a lack of solidity is deemed inconvenient or unaesthetic. Consequently, food producers sometimes resort to a process called hydrogenation. Without going into details, hydrogenation involves the adding of hydrogen to fatty acids—that is, making the fats more saturated and, therefore, firmer.

Margarine is a case in point. Perhaps because it was introduced as a substitute for butter, consumers expected it to be firm like butter. But margarine—at least, some kinds of margarine—is made out of vegetable fats that are high in polyunsaturates. As a result, unless special steps are taken to make it solid, margarine is runny. To produce a firm product, the fat in margarine is hydrogenated. Peanut butter is also frequently hydrogenated so that its fat content will not separate as oil.

Hydrogenation does not eliminate all double bonds: margarine is still less saturated than butter. But if you are looking for foods that are low in saturated fats, it is important to be aware of what is meant by the term "hydrogenated." The margarines that are less hydrogenated—and thus higher in polyunsaturates—are generally softer. Usually they are sold in tubes or tubs rather than as solid blocks. (Some margarines are high in saturated fats even without hydrogenation. These are made out of cheaper vegetable oils such as coconut oil. You should check labels to be sure of what you are getting.)

Cholesterol

Cholesterol is found in virtually all animal cells and plays a vital role in the body's functioning. Although sometimes described as a fatty substance, cholesterol is not, strictly speaking, a fat. It is an alcohol, somewhat like glycerol but thicker.

While cholesterol and fats are distinct substances, the two are usually discussed together, for a sound reason: consumption of fats—the amount and kind—affects the level of cholesterol circulating in the blood. Saturated fats raise blood cholesterol levels, while polyunsaturated fats lower the amount of cholesterol in the blood. Monounsaturates apparently have no impact on cholesterol levels.

As mentioned, the body needs cholesterol to perform some important functions. Among these are the making of strong cell membranes, the formation of adrenal and sex hormones, the provision of protective coverings for certain nerve fibers, and the formation of bile, which is used to digest fats. After the age of six months, however, human beings do not need dietary cholesterol because the body is capable of synthesizing all that it requires from carbohydrates and fats. On average, the liver makes 1,000 mg a day to meet the body's needs. Yet the typical American diet supplies an additional 600 mg of cholesterol a day. (This dietary cholesterol comes from animal foods; vegetable foods do not contain cholesterol, unless it has been artificially added.)

To a degree, the body cuts back internal production of cholesterol in response to dietary intake. This compensatory reduction, however, is apparently only partially effective: high amounts of cholesterol in the diet are usually related to high blood cholesterol levels. This may in part reflect the fact that high-cholesterol foods also tend to be high in saturated fats, which, as discussed earlier, raise blood cholesterol levels. In fact, saturated fats seem to be more responsible than dietary cholesterol for raising blood cholesterol levels.

Blood cholesterol levels have been linked with heart disease and possibly cancer. We will examine the evidence for this link later, but now it is important to point out how cholesterol is carried in the bloodstream. As a lipid, cholesterol is not soluble in water and thus needs to be given a protein coating in order to travel through the blood. There are three principal types of cholesterol-carrying lipoproteins: high-density lipoproteins (HDLs), low-density lipoproteins (LDLs) and very-low-density lipoproteins (VLDLs). The high-density lipoproteins are sometimes called the "good" variety, since they apparently remove cholesterol from the walls of the arteries and return it to the liver, thus retarding the development of atherosclerosis. (It is the deposit of cholesterol and other substances on the walls of the arteries that hinders circulation and promotes atherosclerosis.) The high-density lipoproteins also appear to assist the liver in excreting excess cholesterol through the intestine as bile.

The low-density and very-low-density lipoproteins, on the other hand, have the effect of keeping cholesterol in circulation. As a result, scavenger cells must take on the task of cleansing the blood of excess cholesterol. Some of the scavenger cells end up on artery walls and are thus apparently responsible for the cholesterol deposits that eventually occlude arteries.

In general, about 70 percent of the cholesterol in the blood is of the undesirable kind: low-density and very-low-density lipoproteins. However, the proportions of HDLs and LDLs and VLDLs can be affected by both diet and exercise. While saturated fats in the diet promote cholesterol transport by low-density and very-low-density lipoproteins, a diet high in polyunsaturated fats increases the percentage of high-density lipoproteins. Strenuous exercise also favors production of high-density lipoproteins.

Until menopause, women have a higher percentage of high-density lipoproteins than men of the same age; women also have fewer heart disease problems than men during those years. In most non-human mammals, high-density lipoproteins predominate, a fact that probably explains why carnivores are able to consume so much saturated fat without developing atherosclerosis. A few humans, thanks to genetic good fortune, have high levels of high-density lipoproteins and are thus less prone to developing heart problems.

The Digestion of Fats and Cholesterol

About 50 percent of ingested cholesterol is absorbed; much of it is used to manufacture bile acids in the liver. In the case of fats, the figure is closer to 95 percent for individuals in good health, but insufficient bile, as a result of disease or malnutrition or a plugging of the bile ducts, can cause dietary fats to be excreted.

As it passes down the alimentary tract, fat is broken up by various enzymes. The triglycerides are in general split up into their original components of glycerol and fatty acids, although some triglycerides are not split chemically but simply made into smaller and smaller globules (emulsified). Once the fat molecules and cholesterol are absorbed through the intestinal walls, they are given protein coverings—that is, made into lipoproteins—for their trips through the bloodstream.

Transporting cholesterol to the cells that need it is the main function of the low-density lipoproteins. Usually, a cell that obtains its needed cholesterol from the bloodstream will discontinue its own production of cholesterol. Sometimes, however, a genetic defect will disrupt this self-monitoring or feedback system, with the result that the cell continues to produce cholesterol even though there are ample supplies of it in the blood. This condition has been associated with the early onset of heart disease.

In addition to high-density, low-density and very-low-density lipoproteins, two other lipoproteins deserve mention: chylomicrons, which carry emulsified globules of triglyceride to the liver and fat-storage cells, and lipoproteins formed from fatty acids and the plasma protein albumin. When fat is needed, these albumin-based lipoproteins transport it out of the fat-storage cells.

The glycerol part of a triglyceride is converted into glucose in the liver and then metabolized as a carbohydrate (see Chapter 5). The fatty acids are metabolized mainly in the liver, in a rather complicated process. A dangerous condition known as ketosis can arise if a large amount of fats is ingested during a time when carbohydrate intake is very low. Under normal conditions, the toxic ketones formed in ketosis are broken down into carbon dioxide and water.

The Health Controversy

Are saturated fats and cholesterol bad for us? Do they cause atherosclerosis? Cancer? The concerns are sufficiently compelling to have prompted a U.S. Senate committee to call upon Americans to reduce their average intake of both cholesterol and fats, particularly saturated fats. But, as stated at the beginning of this chapter, controversy is characteristic of this field—another official government body declined to recommend any reduction of either fats or cholesterols in the diet.

Atherosclerosis

Cholesterol has been linked with atherosclerosis (a cause of coronary artery disease). Deposits of cholesterol form part of the substance that clogs arteries. This naturally leads to the conclusion that high levels of cholesterol in the blood promote atherosclerosis. (As pointed out earlier cholesterol that comes in the form of high-density lipoprotein seems to have a benign impact in regard to atherosclerosis, but such cholesterol is generally in the minority in most human beings. Thus, in the following discussion, "cholesterol in the blood" should be taken to mean low-density or very-low-density lipoprotein unless specifically described as high-density lipoprotein.)

The link between high blood cholesterol and heart disease is supported by various studies. The people of Finland have the highest death rate in the world from disease of the coronary artery.

They also have the world's highest percentage of saturated fats in their diet and the highest blood cholesterol levels. By contrast, the Japanese, whose diet is relatively low in saturated fats, have a death rate from coronary disease that is less than one-tenth that of the Finns: 20 per 10,000 over a five-year period compared with 220 per 10,000 for the Finns. The U.S. rate is 185 per 10,000, and the American diet resembles that of the Finns more than that of the Japanese. (A diet that is high in saturated fats, it should be remembered, causes blood cholesterol levels to increase.)

It might be assumed that ethnic groups have different genetic susceptibilities to heart disease, but, at least in most cases, this does not seem to explain the differences in national rates of heart disease. Japanese who move to the United States and adopt diets that are high in saturated fats and cholesterol experience an increase in atherosclerosis. And the same increase in heart disease occurs for other ethnic groups, such as those from Mediterranean countries, who abandon traditional diets that are low in saturated fats.

Hospital observations have yielded similar findings. In a study done in Chicago, the results of which were published in 1981, doctors at three hospitals monitored the health of 1,900 men over a period of 20 years. They found that the men whose diets were lower in saturated fats and cholesterol had a death rate from coronary disease that was one-third below that of the men who consumed large amounts of cholesterol and saturated fats. In Finland two mental hospitals cooperated in a 12-year study in which first one hospital and then the other put patients on a controlled diet designed to lower blood cholesterol through the partial substitution of polyunsaturated fats for saturated fats. During the time when the low-cholesterol diet was in effect at each hospital, the death rate from heart disease declined significantly.

Eggs: Are They a Problem?
A discussion of dietary fats and cholesterol generally does not focus very long on any one food; there are just too many foods for that to be a practical way of proceeding. But there is an exception: eggs. Because of their traditional importance in the American diet as well as their high cholesterol content, eggs merit special consideration.

The yolk of a single large egg has between 250 and 275 mg of cholesterol. Thus, two eggs for breakfast will provide most of the 600 mg of dietary cholesterol that Americans, on average, consume each day. And many nutritionists say 600 mg is far more than should be eaten. But eggs are a good source of important nutrients, particularly protein. Consequently, many people are reluctant to banish eggs from their diets, at least without more evidence than has so far been presented against them.

Different studies have yielded different results. In one experiment, two eggs daily were added to the diets of men hospitalized for heart surgery. After 20 to 54 days, there was no change in the patients' blood cholesterol levels. Another study found a rise in the blood cholesterol levels of older men after one egg daily but a drop when the men consumed two eggs every other day.

These findings have naturally been hailed by egg enthusiasts. However, critics have noted that the diets of the subjects in the studies were not controlled. Among the other shortcomings cited were that no mention was made of what the eggs replaced in the men's diets and that weight changes were not taken into consideration.

Moreover, other studies subject to careful controls have substantiated concern over the impact of eggs on blood cholesterol levels. A study by the Harvard School of Public Health found that patients in a mental hospital who were fed egg yolks experienced an increase in their blood cholesterol levels. An experiment by the National Heart, Lung and Blood Institute revealed that a rise in egg intake disturbed the balance between the different types of cholesterol-carrying lipoproteins in the blood, even if it did not result in an increase in blood cholesterol levels. The study found an increase in a particular type of high-density lipoprotein, designated HDL-c. While most high-density lipoproteins are considered "good" from the viewpoint of atherosclerosis, HDL-c is even more damaging to blood vessels than low-density lipoproteins.

Given the questions that persist about the impact of eggs on blood cholesterol levels, it is probably wise to limit the number consumed.

Cancer

Recent studies have indicated that cancers of the colon, breast and endometrium (the lining of the uterus) may be associated with the same kind of high-fat diet implicated in heart disease. The evidence is not as strong as that pointing to the link with atherosclerosis, but there are grounds for concern.

Some of the evidence stems from experiments with rats. It appears that when cholesterol is added to the diet of rats who already have cancer of the colon, the growth of the cancerous tumors is accelerated. The medium for this effect may be the action of intestinal bacteria. These bacteria produce substances that can cause cancer (or enhance the carcinogenic potential of other substances) as they break down foods that are high in fat and cholesterol. One theory holds that since high-fat meals slow down the digestive process, fecal matter stays in the colon longer than usual, allowing more time for the cancer-causing or -enhancing substances to do damage.

The intestinal bacteria also metabolize cholesterol to produce substances that are similar to female sex hormones. Some argue that such substances could promote cancer in both the breast and the endometrium, since both areas are sensitive to hormones.

Observations of shifting dietary habits and health problems among certain populations also suggest a link between cancer and high-fat diets. Again, the Japanese can be cited as an example. Their traditional diet is quite low in saturated fats, but Japanese who emigrate to the United States and adopt a typically American diet show an increased rate of breast, endometrial and colon cancer. An increase in colon cancer was also seen among Seventh Day Adventists who, at some time in their lives, departed from the sect's traditional vegetarian diet.

Questions about Polyunsaturated Fats

Most of the studies that we have mentioned so far have focused on the harmful effects of saturated fats. Polyunsaturated fats, by contrast, have appeared in a favorable light. Yet some studies have even questioned polyunsaturated fats. A group of Maryland researchers investigating health and dietary records over the past 60 years reported finding no link between cancer and saturated fats, but they did cite a possible connection between hydrogenated vegetable oils and cancer. A study of veterans in Los Angeles who were put on a diet high in polyunsaturated fats found a decrease in deaths from heart disease but an increase in cancer deaths. However, in most cases, the cancer seemed to strike those veterans who did not follow their diet closely. In contrast, several studies of large groups of people showed no increase in cancer risk with higher intakes of polyunsaturates.

Given the conflicting results of such studies—and more could be cited on each side—any link between polyunsaturates and cancer or other health problems appears fairly speculative at this point. It should also be remembered that polyunsaturates have certain positive features: They serve to reduce blood cholesterol levels, for example. And certain polyunsaturates such as those found in soybeans have a substance, known as a protease inhibitor, that may serve to inhibit tumors.

It appears that polyunsaturated fats are preferable to saturated fats. However, that does not mean we should regard polyunsaturates as a panacea, to be added to all foods. Moderation is the watchword. If our overall intake of fats is low, then probably polyunsaturates are good for us, rather than the reverse.

Government Findings

In 1977 the U.S. Senate's Select Committee on Nutrition and Human Needs looked at the evidence linking fats and cholesterol to health problems and concluded that Americans should change their dietary habits. Specifically, the committee recommended that overall fat intake be cut by nearly a third, reducing its proportion to 30 percent of all calories consumed. That 30 percent, the committee said, should be divided evenly, 10 percent apiece, among saturated fats, monounsaturated fats and polyunsaturated fats. Since the average American diet in 1976 included nearly twice as much saturated fat as polyunsaturated fat, the committee was recommending a major change. It also advised cutting dietary cholesterol intake from 600 mg to 300 mg a day.

The Senate panel's recommendations appear to be in line with the numerous studies linking high-cholesterol and high-saturated-fat diets with heart disease, not to mention the possible connection with cancer. Some authorities have recommended even sharper reductions in the consumption of fats and cholesterol. Nevertheless, the committee's recommendations did not go unchallenged. Another government body, the Food and Nutrition Board of the National Academy of Sciences–National Research Council, released a report in 1980 recommending no reduction of fats or cholesterol for the average person. The board stated that no real proof had been presented to show that high blood cholesterol levels caused heart disease or that lowering blood cholesterol would prevent heart attacks. The board went no further than to acknowledge that persons "at risk" should perhaps alter their diets. (This prompted the observation from one of the directors of the famed Framingham Heart Study that "nearly all Americans are at risk [of having] a heart attack.")

The board and others skeptical about the link between heart disease and high-fat diets offer a number of arguments. First, there are always exceptions—persons who eat all the "wrong" foods but never develop heart disease. Then, too, other factors besides fats and cholesterol play a part in the development of heart disease—genetics, stress, physical activity, air pollution, water quality. Why, the skeptics ask, should fats and cholesterol be singled out for blame?

The Bottom Line

While we do not have completely unshakable proof of the connection between heart disease and a diet that is high in saturated fats, there is plenty of strong evidence supporting that theory. As with other health-related controversies, we have to make a decision on the basis of the knowledge available.

A good deal of research indicates that we should cut our intake of cholesterol and fats, especially saturated fats. Some doctors may doubt the need for such a step, but almost none would say it was harmful. In other words, there is nothing to lose from making the recommended dietary changes, and very possibly something can be gained—a longer life.

Some of the specific things we can do to limit our consumption of fats and cholesterol are:

- Cut egg intake to three or four a week.
- Use low-fat or skim milk and milk products.
- Sharply limit consumption of high-cholesterol and high-fat meats, and trim off all visible fat when they are to be eaten.
- Avoid frying and stewing meat, since these cooking methods increase fat content.
- When choosing poultry, select the smaller, younger birds, which have much less fat.
- Avoid whipped toppings and milk/cream substitutes; they contain coconut oil, which is more saturated than butter.
- Eat hard and processed cheeses sparingly. Instead, have cottage cheese, farmer cheese, pot cheese, ricotta or yogurt, particularly the low-fat varieties.

Chapter 4

Carbohydrates

Remember those meals when your father got you to finish your broccoli by threatening to withhold your ice cream dessert?

Remember those snack times when you yearned for some cookies or a hunk of chocolate cake and your mother instead handed you an orange or an apple?

No doubt your parents told you that fruits and vegetables were good for you. They also probably told you that too many sweets would ruin your health. What your parents didn't tell you (if indeed they knew) is that both broccoli and chocolate cake supply the body with chemically related compounds: carbohydrates.

In America's diet-conscious culture, "carbohydrate" is a dirty word. Yet the word covers a vast range of foods: fruits, vegetables, grains and dairy products. In fact, the only noncarbohydrate foods are meat, poultry and fish.

Humankind has been feeding itself with carbohydrates since the dawn of time. In fact, carbohydrates historically have made up most of the food eaten by most of the people in the world. In Asian countries, rice is the principal staple, followed by noodles. Rice and beans form the basis of many Latin American and Caribbean diets. Corn and beans are common foods in Africa. Pasta and rice are basic to the diets of Mediterranean peoples. The potato has long been a favorite of many Europeans. Corn, wheat, potatoes and rice are North American favorites. For centuries bread, the so-called staff of life, has sustained rich and poor in Europe, the Americas, North Africa and the Middle East.

In recent years, however, carbohydrate foods have been spurned as fattening and unhealthy by many in the industrialized nations. Do carbohydrates deserve this tarnished reputation? Let's take a closer look.

What Are Carbohydrates?

Carbohydrates are a group of chemical compounds made up of carbon, hydrogen and oxygen. Plants, using water from the soil and carbon dioxide from the air, produce carbohydrates through the process of photosynthesis. There are generally two atoms of hydrogen for each atom of oxygen (the same ratio as in water), hence the name "carbo*hydrate*."

Carbohydrates are classified according to arrangements of the carbon, hydrogen and oxygen atoms. The smallest, simplest carbohydrates are sugars (monosaccharides and disaccharides). The most complex carbohydrates are starches and fiber, both polysaccharides.

Sugar molecules serve as the building blocks from which all other carbohydrates are constructed (see Chapter 5).

Carbohydrates are further classified according to their digestibility. Sugars and most starches are easily digested and are therefore frequently referred to by nutritionists as "available" carbohydrates. Fiber is difficult, often impossible, to digest. It is therefore termed an "unavailable" carbohydrate.

Many scientists classify fiber as a starch, as both are complex carbohydrates. In chemical structure, fiber is more closely related to starches than to sugars. What chiefly sets them apart are the forms they take in nature and their digestibility.

Some of the most common starches are:

Digestible	Partially Digestible	Indigestible
Amylose	Inulin	Cellulose
Amylopectin		Pectins
Glycogen		Gum
		Mucilage

Sources of Carbohydrates

The simplest carbohydrates are sugars (monosaccharides and disaccharides), and the simplest, most common sugars are glucose and fructose. Both are found in fruits and honey. When a molecule of glucose and another of fructose are bonded, they form the disaccharide sucrose. In its most familiar form, sucrose is used by millions of people as ordinary table sugar, derived from cane or sugar beets.

Glucose is a prime component of most complex carbohydrates (starches). It also circulates in the blood, providing cells with energy. Thus, another name for glucose is "blood sugar."

Starches are found in nature in the seeds, roots and fruit of various plants. Rice, potatoes, wheat and corn are rich in starches. Fiber (also known as roughage or bulk) is derived principally from the hard outer layers of whole grains (i.e., wheat bran) and from tough, stringy plant tissues (cellulose).

Both sugars and starches can be extracted from the foods in which they naturally occur and added to other foods. These so-called refined or processed carbohydrates, removed from their normal source, no longer contain the amounts and varieties of minerals and vitamins they once had. In most instances, refined or processed carbohydrates have little more to offer than calories bereft of nutrients—or *empty calories.*

Are Carbohydrates Necessary?

While high-carbohydrate diets are found around the globe, they are not universal. Eskimos and the Masai people of East Africa, for example, have traditionally subsisted on high-protein, high-fat diets, virtually devoid of carbohydrates.

Few nutritionists would recommend a traditional Eskimo diet, just as few would recommend a diet over-balanced with carbohydrates. Most would agree, however, that carbohydrate consumption is necessary for stable health.

First of all, carbohydrates are an important source of energy. Each gram of carbohydrate provides four calories, the same as in a gram of protein. Moreover, when the body draws upon carbohydrates as its energy source, it spares proteins for their most important functions: building and repairing tissues.

Glucose (blood sugar) guards against the buildup of ketone bodies, or toxic wastes that enter the bloodstream when the body is forced to draw upon fats and protein for energy. At its most extreme, this condition (known as ketosis) can result in brain damage.

Carbohydrates provide the body with carbon molecules needed to make its genetic building blocks: DNA and RNA. Carbon molecules are also bonded into such important compounds as glucuronic acid (needed to detoxify substances in the liver) and galactosides (needed for the proper functioning of the central nervous system).

Digestible carbohydrate foods are the major source of vitamins and minerals. They also add desirable flavorings to diets that would otherwise taste bland.

Indigestible carbohydrates (fiber) lack both available calories and essential nutrients. However, a growing body of evidence points to the importance of fiber in the daily diet. It has been shown that fiber lowers the level of sugar in the blood, which in turn reduces the need for insulin. Under certain circumstances, it can lower the blood level of triglycerides, which have been associated with heart disease.

Certain types of fiber can lower the blood levels of low-density lipids, which are fatty substances considered harmful. By the same token, some types of fiber increase the levels of high-density lipids, which are regarded as beneficial (see Chapter 3).

Fiber stimulates the internal motions of the intestine, speeds up the digestive process and leads to a more regular and complete elimination of solid waste.

Requirements for Carbohydrates

The average American today consumes between 200 grams and 300 grams of carbohydrates a day, yet he or she is probably getting less nutrition per gram than the American of 50 years ago.

In our grandparents' day, bread was a staple at every meal, and more vegetables than meat were seen on the table. Gradually, an increasing portion of the food dollar went for meat and for processed fruits and vegetables. Meals not only became more expensive but actually offered fewer vitamins and minerals.

This trend came to the attention of the U.S. Senate's Select Committee on Nutrition and Human Needs. In 1977, the committee issued revised goals calling for Americans to raise their consumption of complex carbohydrates and naturally occurring sugars from 28 percent of their diets to 48 percent.

A problem faced by the Senate panel then, and a problem that continues today, is that there are no recommended dietary allowances for carbohydrates, as there are for proteins. One reason is that proteins are mostly interchangeable, as long as either separately or together they supply the necessary amino acids. Carbohydrates are much less easy to classify: some are digestible, others are not; some are desirable sources of nutrition, others are not. Since carbohydrates cannot be substituted as readily for one another, it is difficult to say that X number of carbohydrate units is required daily. In addition, more study has been devoted to proteins than to carbohydrates, and therefore, more is known about the relative values of proteins.

Advantages of Carbohydrates ...

As we have seen, carbohydrates are abundant, relatively economical sources of energy and their inclusion in the diet avoids the wasteful, potentially dangerous use of proteins for supplying energy.

The value of complex carbohydrates in the diets of persons with diabetes mellitus is now evident. In the past, diabetics' problems with sugar were regarded as problems with all carbohydrates. Now, however, many diabetics are on low-fat, high-fiber, high-complex-carbohydrate diets. On this regimen some have been able to do entirely without insulin or any other anti-diabetic medication, while others have been able to reduce their insulin requirements. Much of the benefit of fiber for diabetics appears to stem from the fact that when carbohydrates are consumed with fiber, the blood levels of sugar are lower than they are with carbohydrates alone. This, in turn, means that less insulin is required. (For a further discussion of fiber, see Chapter 6.)

You don't have to be diabetic to use the basics of this diet. Many athletes and smart dieters have come to realize that eating foods high in complex carbohydrates can be a pleasant and efficient way to lose weight.

In a study done in 1975, overweight young men who ate high-fiber bread with their meals over a period of eight weeks lost an average of 19.4 pounds. In the same study a similar group who ate a look-alike bread low in fiber dropped an average of 13.7 pounds. These men ate *12 slices of bread daily.* (They could eat anything else they wanted but were required to stay away from highly caloric foods.)

The fact is that bread gives a feeling of being full, thereby helping to reduce the appetite for concentrated-calorie foods, such as cakes and cookies, as well as the total amount of food eaten at each meal. You will note that the weight loss was greater in those who ate high-fiber bread. This is because fiber gives a greater feeling of being full, accelerates the food through the intestinal tract and retains water, producing a larger, softer fecal stool. Fiber adds bulk with few or no calories—certainly a plus for the weight-conscious.

... And Some Drawbacks

Problems related to carbohydrates usually fall into two categories: over-consumption and an inability to digest digestible carbohydrates. One problem is behavioral; the other, medical.

Let's look at the latter problem first.

Digestion begins in the mouth. The enzyme ptyalin helps to break down starches during the chewing process. A deficiency of this enzyme would prevent carbohydrates from entering the stomach in a properly prepared state, hindering digestion.

Persons who have pancreatitis or cystic fibrosis have difficulty with both protein and carbohydrate digestion because of insufficient pancreatic digestive enzymes. The mechanisms of deficiency are different in these two diseases, but the lack of enzymes is a common problem.

Difficulties with absorption in the small intestine—due to excessive internal motions, insufficient motions, lesions of the mucous membrane or failure of endocrine functions—can also interfere with the digestion of carbohydrates.

The problems with over-consumption of carbohydrates generally fall into four categories:

1. Over-consumption of carbohydrates without concomitant under-consumption of other food categories
2. Over-consumption of carbohydrates with concomitant under-consumption of other food categories
3. Over-consumption of refined carbohydrates
4. Over-consumption of indigestible carbohydrates (fiber)

Over-consumption of carbohydrates without a concomitant reduction in the amount of proteins and/or fats consumed results mainly in obesity. Over-consumption of carbohydrates with inadequate consumption of needed proteins and/or fats leads to deficiencies in amino acids and essential body fats as well as obesity. Lack of proteins results in the wasting of lean tissue; lack of dietary fats prevents absorption of fat-soluble vitamins. (For more information on the importance of dietary proteins and fats, see Chapters 2 and 3.)

For many, over-consumption of carbohydrates means over-consumption of empty calories. Besides being self-indulgent, such people are either ignorant or unmindful of proper nutrition. As a result, "junk-food junkies" are shortchanged on vitamins, minerals, proteins and complex carbohydrates. The consequences of these deficiencies include little sustained energy, low resistance to illness, poor skin turgor (the "feel" and elasticity of the skin), lank hair, poor digestion, poor bowel movements and problems with sleeping.

The problems associated with over-consumption of fiber are a different matter. Rather than worrying about what goes into the body, high-fiber dieters are concerned about what comes out. Fiber enables the body to rid itself of many unwanted substances, including toxic materials and possible carcinogens, in a relatively short time because it increases the motion of the bowels. However, this decreased "transit time" (the time it takes food to pass through the body) and the ability of fiber to bind itself to other substances can work to the body's disadvantage. Many minerals, such as calcium, zinc, manganese, iron, phosphorus and copper, may be carried out of the body along with the waste. Other problems related to over-consumption of fiber include a possible loss of vitamin B_{12} and a decrease in the absorption of protein.

Since most well-nourished people consume more than they need of these nutrients, such decreases will be of little consequence, and the situation usually rights itself in a matter of weeks after increasing dietary fiber.

Another problem related to a high-fiber diet—a problem that is relatively minor, although uncomfortable and potentially embarrassing—is the likelihood of an increase in intestinal gas with the initial rise in the consumption of fiber. This is due to the activity of bacteria in the large intestine acting on polysaccharides and causing fermentation. The problem can be minimized by raising the intake of fiber gradually, but it might take several weeks for the intestine to adjust to the increased fiber level.

Selecting Better Sources of Carbohydrates

Although there seems little doubt that fresh fruits and vegetables in season are preferable, from both a nutritional standpoint and a taste standpoint, it is also a fact that processed foods increase the variety as well as the amount of fruits and vegetables available. In addition, there is some question as to whether foods picked while unripe, shipped from afar and stored under perhaps less than optimal conditions offer a better nutritional bargain than foods that are carefully processed. Seasonal variations and regional variations in the nutritive content of these foods must also be taken into account.

There are obviously a number of factors to be considered when making recommendations about which foods to eat. The Select Committee on Nutrition and Human Needs somewhat humbly remarks:

> ... it is important to understand the degree of our ignorance about what constitutes food value. Out of more than 50 known nutrients, Recommended Daily Allowances have been established for only 17. In addition, there is no definitive evidence that food composition described solely in terms of all known nutrients would be an accurate measure of total food value.

Canned produce is thought to retain fewer nutrients than either fresh or frozen foods, though there are times when canned foods may be the better bargain. When food must be stored for a period of time, or when the food is not available either fresh or frozen, canned produce may be best. Much of the food value retained depends on what happens to it in the kitchen. Overcooking produce and/or using large quantities of water in which to cook it tends to lower nutrient value. In any case, it is better to save the water in which produce is cooked and use it in soups, gravies and the like. Thus, even if a significant percentage of the vitamins are in the water, you get them one way or another.

All things considered, it is perhaps best to use both fresh and processed produce to ensure a variety of foods. It is also important to stress the consumption of fresh, raw produce. The traditional lettuce and tomatoes and more common salad greens are fine, but people are increasingly aware that many other foods are also good raw. The salad bar is becoming a welcome addition in many restaurants, and raw foods are being served as appetizers. Cauliflower, broccoli, raw mushrooms, spinach, turnips and garbanzos (ceci beans) add zest and variety. Fresh fruits in season are best served raw, saving the stewed and processed fruits for times when fresh ones are scarcer and more expensive.

Although Americans consume citrus juices in relatively large quantities, in many instances they would do better to *eat* the fruit rather than *drink* it. Most juices do not include any of the pulp, which is a good source of vitamins (as well as bioflavonoids) and fiber. From another point of view, 100 calories of juice are usually not as filling or as satisfying in terms of assuaging hunger as are 100 calories of fruit.

Needless to say, soft drinks and flavor mixes, fruit drinks and drinks flavored with "natural flavorings" offer plenty of carbohydrate calories but few or no nutrients. They are primarily made up of water, artificial colorings and flavorings, and quantities of refined sugar. Such sources of empty calories are advertised to children and adults alike and are of no value to either. One of the problems with these useless high-calorie foods is that they take the place of good foods in the diet. Adding vitamin C to these beverages is even more confusing to some people, who assume that this elevates them to the status of a nutritious food.

Snack foods such as potato chips are also a poor nutritional investment. The Senate Select Committee on Nutrition and Human Needs noted:

> highly refined fruits and vegetables generally should not be viewed as nutritional equivalents or substitutes for the same food in its fresh form . . . . Although it would be possible to restore vitamin C and certain other nutrients through fortification [referring to potato chips versus fresh potatoes] it is doubtful that the numbers and balance of nutrients in the fresh form could ever be duplicated.

Much of the love affair with empty calories has to do with promotion. With some exceptions, there is little promotion of fresh fruits and vegetables. Compare this situation with the advertising of snack and convenience foods in print and on radio and television.

Breads have also been under-consumed in the recent past. Some believe that the "enriched" white breads are nutritionally equivalent to their whole-grain counterparts. Quite aside from texture and taste, which many find inferior to whole-grain breads, enriched white bread has less fiber and, in all likelihood, fewer micronutrients. Although some of the nutrients are restored during "enrichment," there is this concern: Since we are not fully informed about all the nutrients, we may have removed more than we realize from these processed foods, and in restoring the losses, we may be restoring less than we think.

From the standpoint of conserving food resources, it has been argued also that we should rely more on plant than on animal sources to supply part of our protein as well as our carbohydrate and many of our vitamin and mineral needs—a point well taken.

The Bottom Line on Carbohydrates

Carbohydrates are good for us—that is, the complex carbohydrates and the naturally occurring sugars, and at least a moderate amount of dietary fiber. And not only are carbohydrates good for us, but they taste good and serve to fill us both psychologically and physiologically. Carbohydrates provide vitamins and minerals and are efficient sources of energy best suited to the human digestive processes.

A diet high in complex carbohydrates and including a varied selection of fibers can help us to maintain good health as well as become—or stay—slim. Diabetes patients can benefit from this type of diet too. While some of this information is relatively new—and may even seem radical to some readers—revised theories and perhaps even newer conclusions could be only a few months or a few years away.

In the meantime, it may be comforting to know that your parents were right after all: Eat your broccoli. And skip the chocolate cake.

Chapter 5

Sugar

From the standpoint of evolution, a sweet tooth was probably an advantage: It helped our ancestors to pick out the fruits and berries that were ripe and ready to eat. But for the contemporary American, finding enough ripe fruits and berries is not likely to be a problem; getting fat is. And our sweet tooth, satisfied by ever-increasing amounts of sugar, is generally seen as one of the body's most insidious traitors in the struggle against obesity.

Critics of sugar do not limit their indictment to the link with overweight. As a promoter of tooth decay, sugar has long been the chief text of sermons by dentists and parents. Since diabetes mellitus involves a breakdown in the regulation of the body's blood sugar levels, some researchers have argued that a high intake of sugar may play a role in the genesis of this disease. (The weight of opinion, it should be said, holds that it is not the *source* of calories so much as an *excess number* of them that helps cause diabetes.) And a few scientists have even claimed that a high sugar intake is the major dietary cause of diseases of the heart and blood vessels.

This is not to mention the faddists who implicate sugar in everything from hemorrhoids to high crime rates.

On the other side of the argument are those who see sugar as a harmless and good-tasting source of quick energy. "Good nutrition begins with eating," a brochure put out by the Sugar Association says, arguing that people might not eat the foods they should if they were not sweetened.

The debate over sugar is further complicated by the fact that sugar comes in many forms. Some writers have only harsh words for sucrose, the "refined" sugar with which we are all familiar, but are much more positive when discussing honey, for example, or fructose, a sugar found in many fruits. Are such distinctions truly warranted?

That question will be dealt with in this chapter. It will discuss the role of sugar in the American diet and the nutritional implications of that role. What sugar is, how it functions in the body and its possible links to various health problems and diseases will also be put in perspective.

Sugar and Our Diet

The U.S. Department of Agriculture publishes figures on per capita sugar consumption in the United States. The statistics show a relatively stable level of consumption for the past half century, at around 100 pounds a year per person. It appears there has even been a small decline in the last few years.

However, sugar consumption has in fact grown in recent years. The USDA figures cover only refined cane and beet sugar; taking into account the use of corn syrups (which include the sugars glucose and fructose), per capita consumption was 128 pounds a year in 1978. This was up from 122 pounds in 1970. The expanding use of corn sweeteners, encouraged by price hikes for cane sugar, more than made up for the decline in the use of sucrose. Figure 5.1 shows the per capita sugar consumption in the United States from 1962 to 1978.

But when nutritionists voice concern over the growing use of sugar, they are usually thinking of a larger time frame than the past 20 years or 50 years. In 1889 per capita consumption of sugar and syrups was 53 pounds a year—less than half the present level. And in remoter times sugar was even scarcer: A pound of cane sugar in the 13th and 14th centuries cost between one and two shillings in England, or more than a servant received for a week's work. In Elizabethan and Restoration theaters, playgoers who wanted something sweet bought an orange. Nowadays, however, we have solved such problems of scarcity.

Where Does All the Sugar Come From?

Sugar today accounts for nearly a quarter—24 percent—of the

Figure 5.1 *The change in per capita consumption of sugars.*

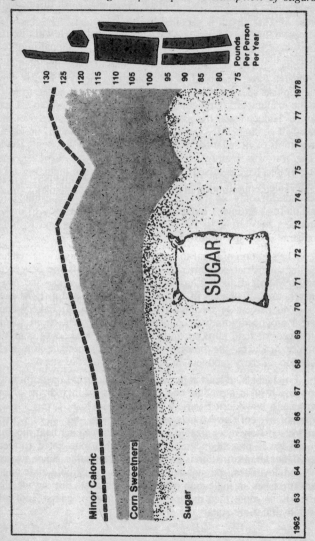

Source: Chris Lecos, "Sugar, How Sweet It Is—And Isn't," *FDA Consumer,* February 1980, pp. 21-23.

calories consumed by an average American. One-eighth of the sugar total—3 percent—comes to us naturally in fruits and vegetables. Another eighth is supplied by dairy products. The rest—18 percent of all the calories we eat—is sugar added to food.

Obviously, a few teaspoonfuls of sugar in one's coffee in the morning cannot account for 18 percent of our total calories (although those teaspoonfuls do mount up quickly). This is why nutritionists speak of "hidden" sugar: sugar that is added to food in the manufacturing process and is consequently likely to escape notice. Hidden sugar has assumed increasing importance over the past half century. Fifty years ago individual consumers purchased two-thirds of all sugar and thus were aware how it was being used. (The rest was mainly used by industry.) Now, however, the proportions have reversed. The food and beverage industries take 65 percent of the refined sugar produced today, while households account for only 24 percent. (The remainder is consumed in institutional settings.) Industry does not use sugar only to make products sweeter; it is also used as a preservative and to hold moisture and improve texture.

The addition of sugar to cereals has become notorious. The leading industrial consumer of sugar, however, is the beverage industry. Soft drink bottlers, together with beer and wine producers, used 26 percent of the refined sugar shipped in 1978 and about 40 percent of the high-fructose corn syrups. Bakery and cereal producers jointly accounted for 13.4 percent of all sugar produced for food purposes in the same year. Makers of confectionery products, the processed food and canning sector, and suppliers of dairy products all use large amounts of sugar.

Food labels, at least at present, offer little help in determining how much sugar a product contains. The list of ingredients often presents a bewildering variety of sugars—sucrose, invert sugar, fruit sugars, corn sweeteners and many others—not all of which are immediately recognizable as sugars. A sweetener near the top of the list is present in greater quantity than one listed further down, but no information is given on actual amounts. Since sugars are carbohydrates, the required information on carbohydrate content furnishes an indication of the sugar content. But the weight listed is no more than an upper limit, since, of course, not all carbohydrates are sugars.

Is There Cause for Concern?

Americans consume far more sugar than they did a hundred years ago and probably more than they are aware of. Does it matter? The government permits sugar to be added to foods in unlimited quantities because it is "generally recognized as safe." Given this sanction, are there solid grounds for all the appeals and injunctions that we wean ourselves from the sugar habit?

Most nutritionists think so. Leaving aside the part sugar plays in tooth decay and obesity (these will be discussed later), there is little that refined sugar has to recommend it besides sweetness and calories, about four per gram. Of course, we certainly need an adequate number of calories to remain in good health, or even to survive. But for most of us, getting enough calories is not the problem. Our concern must be to eat the foods that satisfy our other nutritional needs—for minerals and vitamins, for example—while at the same time giving us the calories we need. The sugar we encounter naturally in fruits and dairy products comes accompanied by these other nutritional values, but as we have seen, this is only a small proportion of the sugar Americans consume. The remainder is largely "empty" calories, sweets that crowd out other, more nutritive foods.

The Chemistry of Sugar

Sugars are a form of carbohydrates, which are in turn a class of chemical compounds made up of carbon, hydrogen and oxygen. Green plants, using water from the soil and carbon dioxide from the air, produce carbohydrates through the process of photosynthesis. Sugars are the smallest and simplest of the carbohydrates; sugar molecules serve as the building blocks out of which other carbohydrates—such as starch—are constructed.

Monosaccharides

The simplest sugars are the monosaccharides. These occur in nature with three to seven carbon atoms, but it is only the hexoses—the six-carbon sugars—that are significant in our diet. As well as being small, by comparison with the other carbohydrate molecules, the monosaccharides are simple in the sense that they cannot be hydrolyzed into smaller compounds. (Hydrolysis involves the splitting of a compound through the addition of a water molecule.)

The most important monosaccharides have the same chemical formula—$C_6H_{12}O_6$—but different properties because the oxygen and hydrogen atoms are bonded to the carbons in different arrangements. These sugars are:

Glucose. Also known as grape sugar, corn sugar and dextrose, glucose is the form of carbohydrate that circulates through the blood; it is the only hexose found in a free state in the fasting human body. (Fasting, here, means a period sufficiently long after a meal for normal digestive processes to have taken place.) Other sugars and complex carbohydrates are in general either broken down into glucose, if it is a constituent, or refashioned into it. Glucose is found in honey, fruits such as grapes and berries, and some vegetables. It is about two-thirds as sweet as sucrose. Starch molecules are made up of chains of glucose, some long and some shorter and branching.

Fructose. Also known as levulose and fruit sugar, fructose is found in a free state in fruits and honey. It is a constituent of sucrose and some complex carbohydrates. Some writers in the past few years have argued that fructose possesses advantages over other sugars for the purposes of losing weight and treating diabetics. These claims will be examined later.

Galactose. Galactose is not found naturally in a free state, but it is a constituent of the sugar found in milk and of some polysaccharides (complex carbohydrates).

Mannose. This sugar is a constituent of certain polysaccharide gums. It is also found in small amounts in several foods, notably manna. Manna is the dried sap of certain plant species, among them the tamarisk tree found in the Sinai desert.

Disaccharides

Disaccharides, or double sugars, are the other main class of sugars: They are composed of two simple sugars (monosaccharides) knitted together with the loss of a water molecule. This gives them the chemical formula $C_{12}H_{22}O_{11}$. The disaccharides break down into simple sugars in the digestive process. The most important disaccharides are:

Sucrose. This is the table sugar obtained from cane and beet with which we are all most familiar. Sucrose consists of a molecule of glucose linked to a molecule of fructose. ("Invert" sugar is a mixture of glucose and fructose obtained by splitting sucrose into its component parts; it is sold in liquid form and used to extend freshness and prevent food shrinkage.)

Lactose. As the name suggests, this is the chief sugar found in the milk of mammals. It is the only carbohydrate of animal origin that has significance for nutrition. The simple sugars galactose and glucose combine to form lactose. Milk contains from 2 percent to 8 percent lactose, depending on the species of animal from which it was obtained.

Maltose. When starch breaks down, as in the malting of barley, it forms the disaccharide maltose, which is composed of two glucose units. Maltose is found in beer and in malted breakfast cereals.

Oligosaccharides and Sorbitol

The monosaccharides and disaccharides comprise the main sugars of interest. The compounds called "*oligo*saccharides" (the prefix means "a few") are, however, also classed as sugars. Some examples of oligosaccharides are the trisaccharide raffinose, found in molasses; and the tetrasaccharide stachyose, which perhaps bears some responsibility for the flatulence caused by eating large amounts of beans.

Sorbitol and similar compounds are closely related to sugars; such compounds are called sugar alcohols. In the case of sorbitol, the aldehyde (CHO) group in a glucose molecule is changed to an alcohol (CH,OH) group. About half as sweet as sucrose, sorbitol is used in products for diabetics because it is absorbed more slowly than sugar and so has less impact on blood sugar levels.

The different sugars (all carbohydrates, in fact) have the same caloric content: about four calories per gram. Figure 5.2 compares the main sugars by sweetness.

How Sugar Functions in the Body

Glucose, the first of the monosaccharides mentioned above, circulates in the blood throughout the body, so that it is present in every cell as a source of energy and for the synthesis of needed substances. The brain, in particular, is dependent upon a steady

FIGURE 5.2 *Relative sweetness of different sugars.*

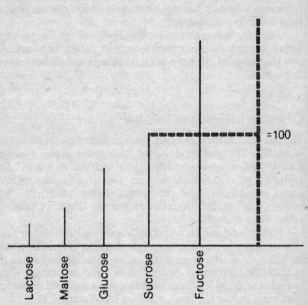

(Sucrose is used to provide a standard of sweetness; i.e., sucrose = 100)

supply of blood sugar (glucose), without which neurological symptoms will soon appear.

It should be emphasized, however, that the vital role glucose plays in the body's functioning does not mean we must be at pains to consume a daily quota of the stuff. The other sugars and the complex carbohydrates furnish an ample supply of glucose, obtained either directly as an end product of the breakdown of disaccharides and polysaccharides or refashioned from other monosaccharides by the liver. The body can also manufacture glucose from the glycerol of fats as well as from certain amino acids. In fact, although nutritionists definitely recommend a balanced diet with a substantial carbohydrate component, it is not clear that carbohydrates are essential to human nutrition. Arctic explorers and certain meat-eating tribes (Eskimos, for example) have remained in good health for extended lengths of time on diets virtually devoid of carbohydrates. However, the metabolism of fats will release dangerous amounts of acids and acetone into the bloodstream unless some carbohydrates are present: The condition is known as ketosis. At least 50 to 100 grams of carbohydrates a day are thought necessary to prevent ketosis and maintain normal metabolic processes. (The diet of most Americans includes 200 to 300 grams of carbohydrates a day.)

Digestion of Sugars

The first stage in the body's utilization of sugar is, of course, digestion. For this, the disaccharides must be broken down into their component hexoses. This occurs in the mucosa of the small intestine, where sucrose, lactose and other double sugars come into contact with splitting enzymes.

If the intestinal mucosa fail to split the disaccharides, because of disease or for genetic reasons, then the sugars will pass on out of the body in watery diarrhea. The enzyme lactase, needed to split lactose, is not produced after childhood by a large number of Asians and some other ethnic groups: Consequently, milk does not play a significant role in their diets.

Once the double sugars have been broken down into monosaccharides, they have to be absorbed through the intestinal wall so they can enter the bloodstream. The villi and microvilli are minuscule projections that greatly enlarge the surface area of the intestine, thus aiding the absorption process. Simple physical diffusion would explain some movement of monosaccharides through the intestinal wall, but in fact they are absorbed at a faster rate than diffusion can account for, and the absorption occurs against a concentration gradient (that is, the monosaccharides move from a less concentrated region to a more concentrated one). The intestine employs what is in effect a chemical pump to transport the monosaccharides into the blood circulation, while in the same process sodium is pumped out. Different sugars compete for this transport mechanism and so have different rates of absorption: Galactose and glucose are absorbed fastest, while fructose and other sugars come through at a slower rate.

Sugar, along with the complex carbohydrates, serves as a fuel for the body: It provides energy to the tissues. But only a portion of the sugar eaten is used immediately as a fuel; some of it is synthesized into glycogen, which serves as a temporary storage reserve, and some is converted into fat. The proportion of carbohydrate, fat and protein in a meal will help determine how much sugar is used immediately as energy and how much is stored, in one form or another. The prior state of the body's energy reserves will also affect the degree to which ingested sugar is expended immediately.

In any case the metabolism of carbohydrates is predominantly the metabolism of glucose. Starch, the key carbohydrate in grains and root plants, is merely a collection of strings of glucose, while sucrose is one part glucose. Other simple sugars entering the body are largely converted into glucose in the liver.

Regulation of Blood Sugar Levels

The liver is the body's chief organ for controlling the level of glucose in the blood. Its regulatory actions are in turn influenced by secretions of hormones from the pancreas and the adrenal, pituitary and thyroid glands.

A person in normal health who has not eaten recently has a blood glucose concentration in the range of 60–85 mg per 100 ml. Eating a meal will increase the concentration to perhaps 140–150 mg per 100 ml, but within a few hours the liver has brought the blood sugar back down to the fasting level. A particularly high level of blood sugar—in the range of 160–180 mg per 100 ml—will result in the excretion of some glucose into the urine. The level at which this occurs varies from one individual to another and is known as the renal threshold for glucose. In healthy individuals the liver controls the glucose level efficiently enough so that excretion rarely occurs, but it can happen if a person has a low renal threshold and eats a meal rich in carbohydrates. A high-starch meal, it should be noted, will have a less sharp impact on blood sugar levels than a high-sugar meal, because of the different rates of absorption into the blood.

A blood sugar concentration above normal is known as *hyperglycemia*; one below normal is called *hypoglycemia*. The first is characteristic of diabetes, and the second is also associated with medical problems. They will be discussed later.

The regulation of blood sugar levels, so important to health, requires a constant balancing act, since glucose in the blood is steadily used up to provide energy to the cells, while it enters through the intestine only intermittently, when we eat. The liver meets this need by reconverting glycogen into glucose.

Glycogen, as mentioned above, is the temporary storage form of glucose. It is sometimes called animal starch, since, like starch from plants, it is made up of immense numbers of chains of glucose units. (Before the synthesis of glycogen from glucose was demonstrated in 1850, by the French scientist Claude Bernard, it had been thought that only plants could perform chemical synthesis.) Some glycogen stores are held in the liver, but most are found in muscle tissue.

Normally the body's glycogen reserve is not great. A walk of two or three hours, if you are not eating as you go, can nearly exhaust the supply. When the glycogen reserves are exhausted, the liver maintains glucose levels by converting protein or fat. About half the amino acids in protein can be used to make glucose, while only about 10 percent of the fat molecule—the glycerol fraction— is convertible into glucose.

Just as the liver has to ensure that sufficient glucose reaches the blood while a person is fasting, so also does it have to arrange for the reduction of the high blood sugar levels following meals. The formation of glycogen for future use removes some glucose from the blood. Since the glycogen store is fairly small—less than a pound for a man of normal size—the amount of glucose that can take this route is limited. Glucose, however, can also form fat, and there is no limit to the amount of fat that can be made. (An experiment with pigs, appropriately, demonstrated this fact: Young pigs put on four times the amount of fat they were fed, showing that it was manufactured from carbohydrates inside the body.) Glucose can also be excreted when the renal threshold is passed, as mentioned earlier, and it contributes the carbohydrate component to a number of important compounds, including DNA and various hormones.

Provision of Energy

And then there is the key function of supplying energy to the billions of cells that compose the body. There are two stages in this process. The first, called glycolysis, or the Embden-Meyerhof pathway (after the men who described it), involves the degradation of glucose to pyruvic and lactic acids. The chemical transformations in this phase occur anaerobically—that is, without requiring oxygen. Each molecule of glucose yields two molecules of adenosine triphosphate (ATP) in glycolysis. The high-energy phosphate bonds of ATP are the form in which energy is transported and made available in the cell.

Further energy is obtained in a second stage, known as the Krebs, or citric acid, cycle. This phase is aerobic (i.e., oxygen is required). The Krebs cycle yields about 15 times as much energy as glycolysis, at the same time releasing carbon dioxide and water.

Glycolysis and the Krebs cycle are classically considered the pathway by which energy is obtained from carbohydrates. However, some studies indicate that a large proportion of the energy supplied by glucose is obtained through its conversion into triglycerides and free fatty acids, which are also burned as fuel by the body.

Several of the processes that remove glucose from the blood are facilitated by insulin, the only hormone known to lower blood sugar. Produced by the islets of Langerhans in the pancreas, insulin helps glucose cross the membrane to enter the cell and also stimulates the production of glycogen and fat. The following are the sources of blood glucose together with its uses and removal mechanisms:

Sources of Glucose	*Ways in Which Glucose Is Removed*
1. Absorption from the intestine	1. Furnishing energy to the cells: (a) glycolysis (b) oxidation via the Krebs cycle
2. Breakdown of glycogen	2. Synthesis of glycogen
3. Conversion of amino acids and fat	3. Conversion into fats
	4. Use in carbohydrate-containing compounds
	5. Urinary excretion

Fructose: A Superior Sugar?

The combination of a national sweet tooth and national diet consciousness produces an unceasing attempt to eat our cake and not have it, too. One consequence of this is the publicity devoted to new or "natural" sugars that are allegedly superior to sucrose. Fructose, in particular, has recently been hailed as an aid in losing weight and as a suitable substitute for glucose for diabetics. While fructose has more to be said for it than many other fad discoveries, neither of these claims has won anything approaching universal endorsement from medical and nutritional authorities.

The argument that fructose will help people lose weight is based on its sweetness: It is about 1.7 times as sweet as sucrose. Because of this greater sweetness, the reasoning runs, people will use less of it. (Fructose has the same number of calories, four per gram, as other sugars, so using as much fructose as sucrose would not provide any savings to a dieter.)

However, skeptics note that fructose's sweetness depends on how it is used. Temperature, acidity and the amount used can all affect the perception of sweetness. In a 1978 study fructose was used in the preparation of sugar cookies, white cake, vanilla pudding and lemonade. With comparisons made on an equal-weight basis, only the lemonade was judged sweeter by the taste panels in the experiment. Furthermore, eating large amounts of fructose—70 to 100 grams in a day—can cause diarrhea.

The alleged benefit of fructose for the diet of diabetics has to do with the claim that its metabolism does not stress the body's insulin system the way glucose does. It is true that fructose is absorbed through the intestinal wall more slowly than glucose and does not require insulin to make its way to the liver; the immediate massive need for insulin created by a glucose-rich meal therefore presumably does not arise. However, many diabetes experts, at least in the United States, feel that these considerations do not in themselves justify classifying fructose as a worthwhile part of a diabetic diet. Long-term studies on the use of fructose as part of a normal diabetic diet still need to be done, according to a review paper by the American Diabetes Association. Skeptics argue that most fructose is converted by the liver to glucose, so that the need for insulin reemerges.

Further, there is concern that a limited endorsement of fructose, holding that it might be acceptable if used in moderation, would be treated by diabetics as wholesale approval. Since fructose is just as caloric as other sugars, and since weight control is of key importance to most diabetics, many doctors have declined to advocate its use, at least pending further study.

Other Much-Touted Sweeteners

Fructose is far from the only sweetener for which great claims have been made. Raw sugar, brown sugar and especially honey are popular with the health-and-natural-food set. They may well be aesthetically superior, but unfortunately, from a nutritional point of view they hold no advantage over sucrose. Raw sugar and brown sugar basically *are* sucrose. Raw sugar is the unrefined product obtained by evaporation of sugarcane juice, while brown sugar is sucrose with a bit of molasses. Honey's composition varies, depending on what nectar is gathered by the bees. Usually, honey is about 15 percent–20 percent water and about 75 percent various sugars, with fructose and glucose the main ones. Gums, enzymes, acids, pollen grains and beeswax also may be found. Some minerals the body needs—potassium, calcium and phosphorus—are present in honey. But the amounts are so slight that honey cannot be considered a useful source of these nutrients—to meet the daily requirement for potassium, you'd have to consume 91 tablespoons of honey, and at that point you would still be less than halfway to reaching the daily quota for calcium and phosphorus, according to a study by the Consumers Union.

Molasses, for a change, does contain some minerals and B vitamins in nutritionally significant amounts. Molasses is the liquid left over after sucrose has been crystallized out of sugarcane or beet juice. It contains a variety of sugars.

Sugar and Health Problems

Americans' large intake of sugar frets nutritionists because, so much of the time, the sugar comes as "empty" calories that provide no contribution (other than energy) to our nutritional needs and make it that much more difficult to balance the rest of the diet. There is not much controversy on this score. But sugar has also been indicted, with varying degrees of plausibility, as a cause of or contributing factor in a number of specific health problems. We will look at these charges now.

Tooth Decay

Of all the ills ascribed to sugar, tooth decay is probably the one people have heard of most. It is also, of all the charges, the most well-founded.

Studies have demonstrated conclusively that populations with diets in which most carbohydrates come in the form of unrefined starches have little tooth decay. A switch to a high-sugar diet, like that of the United States or Western Europe, brings dental problems in its wake.

Dental caries are produced by bacteria in the mouth (mainly Streptococcus mutans) that use sugar as a nutrient. The bacteria metabolize the sugar into a polysaccharide shield that adheres to the teeth (the "plaque" that dentists speak of) and into acids, which eat away tooth enamel.

While sugar thus plays an essential part in tooth decay, the manner in which it is consumed probably matters more than the amount. Sugar that comes in a sticky sweet or in an acid medium, such as a soft drink, is particularly harmful. Sweets eaten between meals are worse than those consumed during meals, when the other foods possibly in some way nullify the effects of the sugar.

An infant can suffer severe tooth decay when a bottle is propped up and allowed to drip into his or her mouth. This condition is known as "nursing bottle syndrome." Milk, juice and sugared water can all cause the decay.

Sucrose, fructose and glucose appear to be equally welcome to and usable by the decay-causing bacteria. Honey, because of its stickiness, poses even greater dangers than other sugary foods.

The measures for preventing decay are well-known to most of us from countless television commercials: Limit sweets, avoid between-meal snacks, and brush and floss the teeth regularly after each meal.

Obesity

Putting on weight is a function of the total number of calories a person consumes, not of the origin of the calories. Some people have claimed that sugar per se promotes obesity, but nutritionists agree that this is not the case.

Nevertheless, the general impression that eating sweets leads to weight gain has more than a little truth to it. One hundred calories of a chocolate bar will not make you fatter than 100 calories of apple, but the chocolate will weigh less, have less bulk and probably leave you hungrier. Consequently, in all likelihood, you will eat more chocolate. Then you *are* taking in extra calories, which, of course, can lead to weight gain.

The addition of sugar to foods raises their calorie total, often markedly, without in general increasing bulk much. As a result, when a person is eating sweets, the feeling of fullness often does not arrive until long after an excessive number of calories have been consumed. A couple of comparisons may make this more apparent. Two ounces of M&Ms have about 275 calories, whereas a pound of apples has only about 260. Four carrots weighing 10 ounces have only 120 calories, less than a half-cup of ice cream (140 calories). And who eats just a half-cup of ice cream?

The apples and carrots, of course, are themselves sweet because of sugars found naturally in them. The point is not that sugar in fruits and vegetables is better because it is in some inscrutable way more "natural" (the sugar in candy bars is "natural," too: It comes from cane or beets), but that fruits and vegetables offer their sugar in a "natural" and healthful proportion to other nutrients.

Sugar's crime is that it makes it so easy to gain weight. This might cause little concern if most of us were slim and fit, but unfortunately, the truth is otherwise. The National Center for Health Statistics, in a study released in 1978, estimated that one-third of the U.S. population was overweight. And it appears that the national health problem has increased in recent years: A study matching adults in 1971–74 with a group of the same height a decade earlier found that both men and women had gained weight. Men and women under 45 were, respectively, 3.8 and 4.7 pounds heavier on average, while those over 45 were an average of 4.8 pounds heavier.

Since sugar's sole nutritional contribution is calories, cutting back on high-sugar sweets is a logical place to start if one is making an effort to lose weight.

Diabetes and Hypoglycemia

Diabetes mellitus and hypoglycemia both involve disorders of the blood sugar level. Diabetes is by far the more common; most instances of hypoglycemia are caused by drugs used to treat diabetes.

Diabetes affects millions of Americans: It is the most common endocrine disease in the United States. The disease is characterized by excessively high blood sugar levels, resulting either from a deficiency of insulin or from the failure of the insulin that is present to perform its normal task of facilitating glucose removal from the blood. Diabetes that develops in middle age (maturity-onset diabetes) is typically of the sort in which insulin is produced by the body but is not effective. In a smaller number of cases, diabetes develops early (juvenile-onset diabetes) and is characterized by a failure of the pancreas to produce insulin.

Nutrition definitely plays a causative role in maturity-onset diabetes. Studies of populations in Japan, Israel and Africa in which dietary patterns have changed show large increases in the incidence of diabetes. Obesity, in particular, is strongly linked with maturity-onset diabetes. Genetic factors are also important: Not all obese persons become diabetic.

Some people have claimed that sugar specifically is a causative factor. They argue that it is a source of repeated stress to the body's insulin mechanism, eventually blunting its efficacy. Several studies have shown that a heightened sugar intake led to an increase in diabetes; however, the increase in sugar was almost always accompanied by an increase in the overall number of calories. In effect, the studies may have only reconfirmed the known connection between obesity and diabetes: A specific link between sugar and diabetes has not been demonstrated. Of course, insofar as sugar contributes to obesity, it can be considered culpable if diabetes develops.

Low-sugar diets are prescribed in the treatment of diabetics, both maturity-onset and juvenile-onset. This is done to prevent excessive swings in blood sugar after meals. Maturity-onset diabetes is at least to an extent reversible through weight loss, so in such cases there is a second reason for limiting sugar consumption.

Juvenile-onset diabetes, it is thought, may be caused by a virus that destroys cells in the pancreas of susceptible individuals. Obesity does not appear to play a role in this disease. Juvenile-onset diabetics are supplied with insulin to make up for the body's deficiency; insulin is sometimes used for maturity-onset diabetes, but in principle the therapeutic aim is to bring about a loss of weight and make the patient's body responsive once more to its internally generated insulin.

Hypoglycemia is not a disease but rather a biochemical mechanism by which a number of diseases can manifest themselves. The overt symptoms of hypoglycemia (low blood sugar) may include weakness, headache and confusion.

Considerable publicity has been given to hypoglycemia, but it is far less common than is sometimes claimed. The most frequent cause is the administration of drugs such as insulin for diabetes. In some other cases hypoglycemia results from the body's own overproduction of insulin after food is digested. There are also instances of hypoglycemia that are not food-stimulated or provoked by drugs.

Eating a sweet with a high sugar content can result in the production of more insulin than is needed, with a resultant drop in blood sugar levels. This is a relatively common occurrence and not to be confused with true hypoglycemia. Sugar apparently does not cause hypoglycemia, but people who suffer from it are put on low-sugar diets for the same reason as diabetics: to prevent sharp swings in blood sugar.

Heart Disease and Atherosclerosis

A few scientists have argued that sugar is a significant cause of heart disease and clogging of the arteries. They cite as evidence some experiments indicating that a high-sugar, low-starch diet results in the production of more triglycerides than a diet with the same overall carbohydrate total but more starch and less sugar. (Triglycerides are a form of fat that has been linked to atherosclerosis.)

The weight of medical opinion, however, holds that fat and cholesterol in the diet are more likely than sugar to contribute to the development of heart disease.

The Reckoning Up

Most of us like to eat sweet foods at least occasionally. Sugar provides the principal means of fulfilling this desire. Unless we practice a particularly unforgiving form of dietary puritanism, we will probably continue to indulge ourselves once in a while.

But this once in a while should be far less often than it is for most Americans today. Sugar, as we have seen, plays an important role *inside* the body, chiefly in the form of glucose, or blood sugar. But from the standpoint of our diet, sugar has no such necessary function. It is simply a source of calories. The glucose and calories we need can be readily obtained from other foods, foods that at the same time will contribute—unlike sugar—to meeting our other nutritional needs. At present, we get 18 percent of our total calories from sugar added to foods, with the result that an extra nutritional burden is imposed on the foods supplying our remaining calories.

Manufacturers of high-sugar sweets have touted them as a source of "quick energy." It is true that the sugar is absorbed quickly into the bloodstream. But that sudden rush of glucose can provoke a counter-response of insulin release that will send blood sugar levels right back down to where they were before the sweet was eaten, or even lower. What we need is good nutrition, not "quick energy."

Apart from tooth decay, sugar does not appear to be directly responsible for major health problems. But there is little doubt that sugar's low bulk and pleasant taste offer an invitation to overeat. And obesity predisposes a person to other health problems.

We consume far more sugar than our ancestors did 100 years ago, and they ate more than their ancestors did. We should strive to reverse the trend and start cutting our intake of sugar.

Chapter 6

Fiber

Today, television commercials promoting breakfast cereals are laced with information about fiber: why it is important, how Brand X stacks up against others in terms of fiber content and so on. Why all the fuss? What started it? Is this just another American dietary fad? Although fiber was "reintroduced" to us in the last decade or so, in fact, it was an integral part of our diet prior to the turn of the century. Then, people thought little about eating potato and apple skins, and so forth; in addition, foods were not refined and processed as they are today. In large part these various refining processes led to the elimination of several sources of dietary fiber. But this, coupled with epidemiological studies on the incidence of colon cancer, diverticulosis, heart disease, etc., led some researchers to examine the dietary changes that have occurred over the last 50 years or so in order to determine whether or not these changes could be responsible, to some degree, for the disease patterns that have emerged in the United States during that time period.

What Is Fiber?

Remember your mother peeling apples, potatoes, pears, etc., to remove the skins before making a variety of pies or boiled potatoes? Unfortunately, all those skins she peeled off were excellent sources of dietary fiber for you! Raw vegetables and fruits contain a lot of fiber; so do whole-grain breads, muffins and cereal products. Rolled oats are another good source of fiber.

What does this fiber consist of? Simply stated, fiber is indigestible plant material. These indigestible carbohydrates, such as pectin, cellulose and other substances, make up the cell walls of plants. This part of fruits and vegetables is often referred to as "bulk" or "roughage." It is only present in plant sources; it does not supply any nutrients whatsoever; and it is not absorbed by the body.

Why Is Fiber Important?

In light of the fact that it has no nutritional value and is not absorbed by the body, one might easily wonder why dietary fiber is necessary at all. Although fiber passes through the digestive tract virtually unchanged, it is very important in the digestive process because it provides bulk to the stool; in addition, most types of dietary fiber have a high water-absorbing ability. In particular, this affects intestinal transit time—in other words, the amount of time it takes for foodstuffs to pass through the intestinal tract. When foods don't pass through the digestive system at normal rates, a variety of problems may ensue: constipation, hemorrhoids, diverticulosis—even cancer of the colon and rectum have been linked to lack of dietary fiber.

What Happened to Fiber?

The Industrial Revolution rapidly transformed this country from miles and miles of farmland into rows and rows of cinder block houses, paved streets and whistling factories. In the process, the way we lived—and the way we ate—also changed. The days of growing your own vegetables and fruits quickly disappeared for most, to be replaced by corner fruit and vegetable stands and, ultimately, the supermarket. Of course, part of what makes it possible for supermarkets to even exist are the technological changes in food processing that occurred in the first half of this century. Sophisticated methods of refining foods and "preserving" them make it feasible for mass quantities to be shipped across the country and maintained or stored until sale. Unfortunately, however, some of these "refining" processes result in stripping the breads and vegetables of many of their natural elements.

Over a century ago, for example, new methods of milling resulted in virtually eliminating all the fiber from bread. Giant rollers were used to crush grain, and in the process, the germ (the most nutritious part of the seed) popped out. What was left to process was the starchy carbohydrate portion of the grain. Flour made in this new way did not spoil as quickly. Further improvements were made in the refining process, and what we now know as fine-grain white bread was born. Little did we realize, however, that in the process the nutritional elements of the grain were eliminated (although bread manufacturers subsequently fortified their products), as were the fibrous elements.

There were some who recognized what was happening to our diet almost immediately; in 1920, for instance, Dr. John H. Kellogg (of Kellogg cereals) advocated a regular diet of fresh fruits, vegetables and cereals to combat constipation and other such complaints. But his extolling the importance of dietary fiber, along with some others who took the same stand, was not enough to counteract the massive dietary changes that were sweeping this country and other Western countries as well. Another 50 years passed before investigators began again to take a hard look at the role of fiber in the diet. Once they did, they soon discovered that all of the refining and processing was in some respects a double-edged sword: Yes, it enabled millions to receive foods from different parts of the country and brought other benefits, and the newer methods of milling did improve the life of flour, but in the process some nutrients and fiber were lost, and it seemed that this was taking its toll in a number of ways.

The Role of Fiber in Disease Prevention

Dr. Denis P. Burkitt, a British physician, spent approximately 20 years studying disease patterns among rural Africans. In his work Dr. Burkitt noted that cancer of the colon and rectum was almost unknown among these peoples, who consumed a diet high in fiber. Dr. Burkitt recognized that the incidence of these two types of cancer in particular had risen considerably in the last few decades; he hypothesized that perhaps the elimination of fiber from the diet was a contributing factor.

To test this hypothesis, Dr. Burkitt and his colleagues compared the intestinal transit times and the differences in bowel movements of the rural Africans with those of Westerners. Overall, they found that the Africans had relatively easy, frequent bowel movements, whereas people in Western countries had more infrequent and difficult bowel movements. They also found that intestinal transit time for the rural Africans averaged 36 hours, compared to an average of 77 hours for British men who consumed a diet low in fiber. The researchers subsequently observed that diseases such as colon and rectal cancer, and diverticulitis and appendicitis were far more common among Western populations than among the Africans.

Of course, it was still unclear just what fiber did to apparently help protect the Africans from these digestive disorders. Dr. Burkitt continued his studies and later reported that those who eat a low-fiber diet, which is so common among Western peoples, may have bacteria in the colon that turn normal bile salts (which are excreted into the colon *after* the bile has performed its digestive functions) into cancer-causing substances. Dr. Burkitt's research sparked a controversy and led other research teams to consider the significance of dietary fiber in the prevention of disease.

Let's take a closer look at a few of the health problems in which a low-fiber diet has been implicated and what effects an increase in dietary fiber can have on such disorders.

Constipation and Hemorrhoids

Few would argue that constipation and hemorrhoids are among our most common complaints. Today more than 700 laxatives are on the market, and it's a safe bet that few medicine cabinets in the United States are without some kind of laxative preparation. Interestingly enough, laxatives can actually *cause* constipation; their chronic use results in the colon's becoming dependent on them, and ultimately, the colon has difficulty acting on its own to propel the waste products through the colon and to the rectum for excretion.

Constipation can generally be avoided by proper dietary measures; this includes an appropriate intake of fluids daily and a reasonable intake of dietary fiber. Regular exercise also helps to maintain bowel regularity.

Hemorrhoids may also be attributed to a lack of dietary fiber. Essentially, hemorrhoids are varicose veins; the hemorrhoidal veins are situated in the anal canal and the walls of the rectum. Constant straining at stool can result in the development of hemorrhoids because the anal canal and the walls of the rectum become irritated. The most common types of hemorrhoids, in fact, are attributable to chronic constipation.

Since a high-fiber diet can eliminate the problem of constipation, and hemorrhoids often go hand in hand with constipation, a high-fiber diet can go a long way to alleviate both these chronic problems.

Colon and Rectal Cancer

Studies to date do not prove that colon and rectal cancer are unquestionably due to a lack of dietary fiber; however, there is evidence to show that countries that consume high-fiber diets have a strikingly lower incidence of these cancers. This statistical association suggests that fiber plays some role in the prevention of colon and rectal cancer. Of course, it is also true that stresses of modern life, coupled with other dietary changes, may contribute to the development of these cancers; but it certainly makes sense to eliminate risk factors, such as a low-fiber diet, that have been linked to these diseases. In this case, in particular, *adding* fiber to the diet does not require any major change in life-style; in fact, it is generally *less* trouble to leave the fiber on (apple skins, potato skins) and to eat vegetables raw and unpeeled. This saves preparation time. About the only change we have to make is to switch from refined white breads to whole-grain breads and muffins.

Diverticular Disease

Diverticulosis is an "outpouching" of the intestinal wall. Diverticula are present throughout the intestinal walls and don't present any problem until they become inflamed (diverticulitis). For years this problem was treated by a bland diet, but new evidence suggests that coarse bran is a more effective therapy. Why? Again, for years it had been assumed that low-fiber, bland diets were needed to "rest" the colon, but in fact, these bland diets actually resulted in the colon's working harder to propel a small, hard fecal mass through the intestine. High-fiber diets, on the other hand, add bulk to the stool and result in smoother and faster intestinal transit.

Obesity

With respect to obesity, just a few simple observations will help to clarify the contribution dietary fiber can make. The incidence of obesity is extremely high in this country, where sugar substitutes, refined foodstuffs, etc. are available in abundance. On the other hand, obesity is uncommon in countries where the diet is primarily made up of starchy carbohydrates with the natural fiber intact. Fiber absorbs water and adds bulk; as such, we are far less likely to overeat. Fibrous foods also take longer to eat because more chewing is involved.

Heart Disease and Diabetes

The role of diet in coronary disease has been explored for decades. Hundreds of researchers have studied the relationship of dietary fats and cholesterol to the development of atherosclerosis (fatty deposits in the arteries). How can fiber help? Certain kinds of dietary fiber, such as the fiber found in rolled oats, guar gum (found in beans) and pectins (found in most fruits), can help to lower serum cholesterol levels significantly. Specifically, one study carried out at the Veterans Administration Hospital in Lexington, Kentucky showed that long-term treatment with a high-fiber diet helped to reduce the level of low-density lipoproteins (LDLs are a cholesterol fraction that has been identified as harmful when present in the blood in high amounts) and increased the level of a beneficial lipoprotein, called high-density lipoprotein (HDL).

Recent work also indicates that diabetics fed high-fiber diets may be able to eliminate anti-diabetic medications or insulin because of the effects the fiber has on blood sugar levels.

Putting Fiber Back in Our Diet

The steps we should take to reintroduce fiber into our diet are simple. To begin, we should look for breads and cereals and muffins that say "whole grain" on the label. Cereal labels may say "rolled oats," and both bread and cereal labels may say "whole wheat."

Raw fruits and vegetables contain more fiber than refined and pureed ones. Salads with lots of unpeeled tomato slices and unpeeled cucumber and zucchini slices also add to dietary fiber intake (see table 6.1).

It is difficult to say just how much fiber a day you need, but a reasonable guideline is to substitute a number of whole-wheat and whole-grain products and more fresh fruits and vegetables for the processed sugars and animal fats you are now eating.

Finally, it should be pointed out that fiber, like anything we eat, can also be overdone. Too much fiber, for example, can cause intestinal gas, and a diet very high in fiber can end up carrying out of the body certain nutrients, such as calcium, magnesium and vitamin B_{12}. For most who are currently consuming a low-fiber diet, simple substitutions of high-fiber products will ensure a safe and adequate dietary intake of fiber.

TABLE 6.1
FIBER IN SELECTED FOODS

Food*		Fiber (mg)
Almonds	1 cup	3.85
Apples	1 med.	1.8
Artichokes	1 avg.	2.4
Asparagus	1 cup	.945
Avocados	1 avg.	3.2
Beans, Baby Lima	1 cup	3.0
Beans, Snap	1 cup	1.2
Beans, White & Red	1 cup	3.0
Blackberries	1 cup	5.9
Blueberries	1 cup	2.2
Bran (all-bran)	1 cup	.42
Breads		
Cracked Wheat	1 slice	.1
Pumpernickel	1 slice	.4
Rye	1 slice	.1
Whole-Wheat	1 slice	.4
Broccoli	1 cup	2.0
Brussel Sprouts	1 cup	2.1
Cabbage	1 cup	1.0
Carrots	1 cup	1.5
Cashew Nuts	1 cup	1.96
Chestnuts	1 cup	1.66
Coconut	1 cup	2.7
Corn	1 cup	1.1
Farina	1 cup	.2
Lentils	1 cup	2.4
Honeydew Melon	2″ wide	.9
Oatmeal	1 cup	.5
Parsley (raw)	1 cup	.9
Parsnips	1 cup	3.0
Peanuts (roasted)	1 cup	3.89
Pears	1 avg.	2.8
Peas	1 cup	3.2
Peppers (raw)	1 cup	1.12
Plums	2 med.	.4
Popcorn	1 cup	.3
Potatoes (baked in skin)	1 lg.	1.2

TABLE 6.1
FIBER IN SELECTED FOODS

Food		Fiber (mg)
Potatoes (Frenchfried)	10 pieces	.5
Prunes	1 cup	2.2
Radishes (raw)	1	1.4
Raisins	1 cup	1.4
Raspberries (black)	1 cup	7.65
Rice (puffed)	1 cup	.1
Squashes	1 cup	1.1
Soybean Sprouts (raw)	1 cup	2.3
Tomatoes	1 cup	.8
Turnips	1 cup	1.15
Walnuts	1 cup	2.13
Wheat (puffed)	1 cup	.2

*Figures given are for raw fruits and cooked vegetables unless indicated.
Source: U.S. Department of Agriculture, Agriculture Handbook No. 456.

Chapter 7

Vitamins

In the past few years, there has been a great cry about vitamins. Many knowledgeable people claim that if we would only eat sensibly, we would automatically receive all the vitamins we need. Others insist that a number of our current ailments are due to vitamin deficiencies, which could be eliminated by taking extra vitamins, eating special diets, avoiding certain foods, etc. No wonder most people are confused.

The truth is that for healthy people vitamin needs can be supplied by a balanced diet. If for some reason an individual is not getting all the required amounts of vitamins from his or her diet, then—with professional guidance—vitamin supplements can be taken to make up for deficiencies as indicated.

The major problem is to determine whether you really need a vitamin supplement or whether you're being swayed by the extravagant claims and misconceptions surrounding vitamins and vitamin supplements. If you feel that you're not getting the proper amount of vitamins despite a balanced diet, then consult your physician. He or she can help determine what you lack and how best it can be supplied. If you have doubts about the adequacy of your diet, consult a professionally trained nutritionist or your doctor.

If it is important to establish what vitamins are and what they can do for us, it is just as important to establish what they are not and what they cannot do for us.

What Are Vitamins?

The name *vitamine* was coined by Casimir Funk in 1912. He was a Polish scientist working at the Lister Institute in London and engaged in research on some of the major maladies of the time—rickets, scurvy, beri-beri and pellagra. Although many researchers were investigating these same disorders, there was little agreement as to their cause. The then recently evolved theory of germs as causative agents of disease led many to believe that these widespread diseases, too, were contagious, but researchers had been unable to demonstrate an infectious agent. Based on the combined findings of many of these investigators, Funk formulated the idea that some food deficiency must lie at the root of all of these diseases. Although the existence of carbohydrates and fats was known, the possibility of other nutrients had not been suspected. Funk suggested that some unknown substances must exist that were necessary for life (hence, "vita") and that they belonged to the "amine" class. His first supposition was correct, although he was mistaken about the second, since most of the vitamins do not belong to the amine group.

Although Funk's theory sparked a flurry of research to isolate and identify these new nutrients, and many *were* identified, the search still continues. Vitamins are now known to be organic compounds required in small, but *significant* amounts to support and maintain life. Most of these vitamins must be supplied by outside sources, although some may be made in the intestine by bacteria normally found there.

In addition to appearing as natural constituents of foods, vitamins are also available as manufactured chemical substances and as "natural" vitamins—each in a variety of forms: powders, pills, capsules and liquids. Guidelines for selecting the appropriate supplement—if needed—appear in the section "Vitamin Supplements."

At present it is generally conceded that 13 of these micronutrients that have been identified are necessary to sustain life. Additional substances, some of which may or may not be vitamins and may or may not be necessary for life, are undergoing investigation. One cannot be dogmatic about the importance of these latter substances, since today's certainty may be tomorrow's error, as has been proved many times in the past.

What Do Vitamins Do?

Vitamins are essentially regulatory substances that control the innumerable phases of fat, protein and carbohydrate digestion. In these roles they form hormones or act with other substances to form enzymes. They also form complexes with proteins. One such example is vitamin A, which joins with protein to help form part of the visual pigment enabling us to see.

Virtually every biochemical action in the body involves one or another vitamin. Every action we perform requires the presence of vitamins, as does every action of our cells within the body. In conjunction with amino acids, vitamins and minerals control cell respiration, without which life cannot continue. Less than optimal concentrations of any of these vital nutrients permit less and less effective cell respiration, but absence of any will eventually cause cell death. And since we are made up of cells, their individual fate becomes our own.

Measuring the Micronutrients

As is suggested by the designation *micronutrient*, very minuscule quantities of these substances are required. It has been said that the amount of vitamins a person requires for an entire year would fit comfortably inside a thimble! But don't let the minute quantity deceive you as to their importance. How, you may ask, can such tiny quantities be measured?

Briefly, there are two ways to measure vitamins—chemically by weight and biologically by IUs (international units). The biological method is usually used first until as much as possible has been determined about the vitamin. This method involves using different species of animals to test different vitamins, depending on which animals require outside (or "exogenous") sources of the vitamin in a manner similar to that of humans. In such a study a number of animals are fed a diet that is adequate to fill their nutritional needs except for food containing the one vitamin that is being studied. When the animals display lack of growth or a symptom of deficiency appears, the vitamin under study is then given until the symptoms are reversed. The amounts required to reverse the symptoms are measured by units. The actual name of the unit is often that of the researcher. The *international unit* designation is simply an attempt to use standardized terminology.

The latest U.S. government tables report the requirements for the fat-soluble vitamins D and E in international units and the requirements for the fat-soluble vitamin A both in international units and as retinol equivalents (the weight of preformed vitamin A). The other fat-soluble vitamin, K, was the last fat-soluble vitamin discovered. Although exact requirements for vitamin K have not been defined, recommended quantities for daily consumption have been agreed upon. These are listed in the 1980

RDAs and are measured by weight, as are the requirements for water-soluble vitamins.

The chemical methods of measuring vitamins differ for each vitamin. Because the amounts involved are so minuscule, ordinary extracting and measuring techniques are out of the question. For example, the amount of thiamine (vitamin B_1) in an entire cupful of wheat is about 1/56,000 of an ounce. Although the chemical methods are much less expensive and require much less time, they may be less accurate than biological methods. In the event of any discrepancy between biological and chemical results, the former are chosen as standards.

Naturally, animal studies do not necessarily indicate that exactly the same findings will apply to humans, although animal testing has proved to be quite predictive. There are vast differences between men, women, children of various ages, older people and people in different physiologic states (pregnancy, lactation, illness, athletic training, etc.), just as there are vast differences in climate, level of physical activity and perhaps other factors that will alter vitamin requirements. In addition, it must be remembered that the amounts of any nutrient necessary to prevent manifest signs of deficiency are quite different from the amounts that should be present to ensure optimal health. Indeed, it is questionable whether the latter quantities have been determined—an issue that will be addressed later.

You will notice that the table appearing in the appendix that lists vitamins available in foods follow the same system used for nutrients in the RDA listing. So for all practical purposes, as long as the daily requirements and the amounts available are expressed in the same measurements, it can be relatively easy to figure out if your diet provides sufficient quantities of nutrients. Hence, despite complex measuring techniques, one need not be a chemist to understand vitamin needs.

Fat-Soluble Vitamins

All of the fat-soluble vitamins must be dissolved in fat before they can be absorbed into the bloodstream through the walls of the intestine. Bile, produced by the liver, and fatty acids are required as solvents to aid in this process. Therefore, persons with low dietary fats and/or liver problems may not be able to absorb enough of these vitamins.

Vitamin A (Retinol)

Sources

- Only *animal sources* (whole milk, eggs and liver) contain preformed vitamin A. The more protein taken in the diet, the more vitamin A is required.
- *Plant sources* of carotenoids (substances found in plants that the body needs to make vitamin A), which are converted into vitamin A by intestinal cells, include dark green and orange vegetables (carrots, pumpkins, yams, apricots, broccoli, parsley, cantaloupe), corn, soybeans, tomatoes and palm oil.

Functions

- Combines with proteins to make visual pigments for both day and night vision.
- Required for growth and repair of all cell membranes (with vitamin E).
- Required for the health of the eye itself, the skin and mucous membranes throughout the body.
- Essential for protein metabolism in the liver.
- Acts as a coenzyme in the skin, the bone, the retina and the liver and adrenal glands.
- Helps form infants' bones and teeth.
- Essential for glycogen synthesis.
- Regulates formation of cartilage.
- Regulates synthesis of some hormones.
- Aids in maintaining health of the reproductive system.
- May aid in the synthesis of RNA and the absorption of RNA in the liver.

Symptoms of Deficiency

- Night blindness (difficulty in seeing in dim light) is an early sign. Dry eyes and lack of pigments lead to blindness later.
- Rough, dry skin.
- Growth retardation in children due to impaired metabolism of hormones, skeletal tissue and membranes.
- Increased susceptibility to infections due to damage to the linings of the lungs, gastrointestinal tract, salivary glands and tear ducts.
- Deficiency of vitamin A leads to losses of vitamin C, with its associated symptoms.

RDA

Infants: birth to 6 months	420 μg* RE
6 months to 1 year	400 μg RE
Children: 1–3 years	400 μg RE
4–6 years	500 μg RE
7–10 years	700 μg RE
Males: 11 years and over	1,000 μg RE
Females: 11 years and over	800 μg RE
Pregnant women	an *extra* 200 μg RE
Lactating women	an *extra* 400 μg RE

*μg = micrograms

Toxic Level

Prolonged ingestion of more than 15,000 RE (50,000 IU) daily can result in symptoms. In children and infants, even one excessively high dose can cause symptoms.

Symptoms of Toxicity

- In infants—transient hydrocephalus (an accumulation of cerebrospinal fluid within the skull; condition may cause convulsions) and vomiting.
- In older people—lethargy; profuse sweating; headache; abdominal pain; bone and joint pain; brittle hair and nails; irregular menses; peripheral edema; dry, scaly, rough skin; exophthalmos (protruding eyeballs).

Vitamin D (Calciferol, Cholecalciferol and Ergocalciferol)

Also acts as a hormone with calcium.

Sources

- Oils (cholesterol) normally present on the skin convert to vitamin D in the presence of sunlight or ultraviolet light from any source and are then absorbed.
- Animal sources are fish liver oils (cod, turbot, halibut); butter; egg yolks; fortified milk; fortified margarine; fatty fishes and crustaceans such as tuna, salmon and shrimp.

Functions

- Regulates proper bone growth and repair.
- Maintains hardness of the teeth and bones.
- Helps maintain proper calcium and phosphorus balance in the body along with the parathyroid hormones.

- Acts as a coenzyme in bone, liver, kidney and intestinal metabolism.

Symptoms of Deficiency
- In children deficiency causes rickets, a disease characterized by deformed bones and retarded growth, as well as soft teeth.
- In adults spontaneous fractures can result from softened bones, and decayed teeth are common.
- Reduction in parathyroid activity results in secondary deficiencies.
- Diminished kidney function.
- Reduced muscle tone.

RDA*

Infants and children: birth to 10 years	10 µg
Males: 11 years and over	1,000 µg
Females: 11 years and over	800 µg
Pregnant or lactating women	an *extra* 5 µg

*10 µg cholecalciferol (the naturally occurring vitamin D in animal tissues) equals 400 IU of vitamin D.

Toxic Level
For infants 3,000 IU.
For adults 1,000 IU per pound per day.

Symptoms of Toxicity
- Early symptoms in children include excessive thirst, excessive urination, lack of appetite and vomiting.
- Infant hypercalcemia (an excess of calcium) with calcification of kidneys, blood vessels and deposits of calcium in the skin can result from excessive intake that may be related to food fortification. Generally, this only occurs in cases where highly fortified foods are eaten in excess and to the exclusion of others.
- Similar symptoms can occur in adults.

Vitamin E (Tocopherol)

There are eight forms of tocopherol, of which alpha-tocopherol is the most active.

Sources
- Plant sources such as soybean, cottonseed and corn oils are

rich in vitamin E. *Only* plants can produce the vitamin.
- Fruits, vegetables and whole-grain products provide varying amounts.
- Meats, eggs and dairy products are relatively poor sources.

Functions

- Vitamin E acts primarily to protect polyunsaturated fatty acids, other fat-soluble vitamins and vitamin C from being oxidized; it also helps integrate vegetable oils into cellular and tissue membranes.
- Essential for the functioning of nervous, digestive, excretory, circulatory and respiratory systems because it helps in maintaining cell membranes.
- Protects the body from pollutants and poisons created by the breakdown of organic substances.
- Promotes normal growth patterns and proper development of muscle tissue throughout the body.
- Aids the body in responding to stress.
- Has little or no effect on sexual function in humans but helps maintain the reproductive system in laboratory animals.
- Is a detoxifying agent and prevents oxidation; it is thought that this may aid in preventing or slowing the aging of cells and tissues.

Symptoms of Deficiency

- There are no clinical depletion symptoms; however, because of cell membrane protection of red blood cells that is provided by vitamin E, it can help prevent certain types of anemia.
- Induced deficiencies in laboratory animals result in a number of disorders related to the level of polyunsaturated fatty acids in the diet. There is a general lack of functioning or poor functioning of the reproductive system involving male and female animals and their young. In the muscular system there is a type of muscular dystrophy, and in the nervous system there are lesions that may be related to the muscular symptoms. *Red blood cells* do not survive as long as normal.

RDA

Infants:	birth to 6 months	3 mg
	6 months to 1 year	4 mg

Children: 1–3 years	5 mg
4–6 years	6 mg
7–10 years	7 mg
Males: 11–14 years	8 mg
15 years and over	10 mg
Females: 11 years and over	8 mg
Pregnant women	an *extra* 2 mg
Lactating women	an *extra* 3 mg

Toxic Level
Because only minute quantities can be stored in the body, there is virtually no chance for toxic levels to build up. Vitamin E is thought to be the least toxic of all the vitamins.

Symptoms of Toxicity
Not seen. Very extreme levels of supplementation may increase blood pressure.

Vitamin K (Coagulation Vitamin)

Sources
Organisms in the intestine produce the vitamin from:
- *Animal foods*—pork and beef.
- *Plant foods*—dark green leafy vegetables, cauliflower, tomatoes, peas and carrots.

Functions
- Acts as a coenzyme required for protein clotting factors in the blood.
- Is a liver coenzyme for energy metabolism and respiration.

Symptoms of Deficiency
A tendency to bleed or outright hemorrhaging.

RDA not established.
Figures represent safe and adequate daily intakes.

Infants: birth to 6 months	12 μg
6 months to 1 year	10–20 μg
Children: 1–3 years	15–30 μg
4–6 years	20–40 μg
7–10 years	30–60 μg
Males: 11–18 years	50–100 μg
19 years and over	70–140 μg

| Females: 11–18 years | 50–100 μg |
| 19 years and over (including pregnant or lactating women) | 70–140 μg |

Toxic Level
None known. Possibility is remote because of the body's limited capacity for storage of vitamin K.

Symptoms of Toxicity
Extremely high doses of a synthetic form of vitamin K have caused yellow skin coloring in low-birth-weight babies, probably due to increased breakdown of red blood cells.

Water-Soluble Vitamins

There are 9 vitamin B complex vitamins and vitamin C that make up the 10 currently recognized vital water-soluble nutrients. Because these vitamins act together most of the time and are frequently found together in the same foods, it is important to consider them together in terms of adequacy of intake. Often the absence or relative inadequacy of one or more will prevent adequate functioning of the remainder in various processes of metabolism.

As a group, these water-soluble vitamins are more fragile than fat-soluble vitamins and are more readily destroyed by improper food preparation, exposure to heat and light, and various means of processing.

Vitamin B₁ (Thiamine)

Sources
- *Animal foods*—beef kidney, lean pork and ham, eggs.
- *Plant foods*—brewer's yeast, wheat germ, whole-grain products, plums, prunes, raisins, legumes and green vegetables.

Functions
- An essential coenzyme for all cells; needed to release energy from carbohydrates.
- Aids in the synthesis of the hormone (acetylcholine) that transmits impulses from one nerve cell to another.
- Acts as a coenzyme in certain liver functions.

- Assists in growth and repair of tissues.
- Aids in maintaining health of heart, nerve, muscle and digestive tissues.

Symptoms of Deficiency

- Those affecting the gastrointestinal tract are poor appetite, poor digestion and constipation, and weight loss.
- Those affecting the central nervous system are poor reflexes, weakness, irritability and loss of memory, depression and psychosis.
- Those affecting the cardiovascular system are "palpitations," rapid heartbeat with small amounts of exertion, chest pain, very low blood pressure, distended veins and bluish skin color due to lack of oxygen (cyanosis).
- The milder symptoms occur before clinical beri-beri is evident. Beri-beri may occur in the wet form (swelling of the tissues) or the dry form (mostly disorders of movement and mental symptoms).

RDA

Infants: birth to 6 months	0.3 mg
6 months to 1 year	0.5 mg
Children: 1–3 years	0.7 mg
4–6 years	0.9 mg
7–10 years	1.2 mg
Males: 11–18 years	1.4 mg
19–22 years	1.5 mg
23–50 years	1.4 mg
51 years and over	1.2 mg
Females: 11–22 years	1.1 mg
23 years and over	1.0 mg
Pregnant women	an *extra* 0.4 mg
Lactating women	an *extra* 0.5 mg

Toxic Level

None known for oral form. Some patients develop a sensitivity after multiple thiamine injections.

Symptoms of Toxicity

See "Toxic Level." Individual sensitivity reactions have been noted but no real toxicity.

Vitamin B₂ (Riboflavin)

Sources
- *Animal foods*—organ meats (heart, liver, kidneys) of beef, veal, pork and lamb or mutton; meats in general; eggs and all dairy products; salmon.
- *Plant foods*—yeast; whole grains; dark green leafy vegetables, particularly broccoli.

Functions
- Works with vitamin A to maintain health of mucous membranes throughout the body and helps preserve the health of the skin, eyes and nervous system.
- Acts as a coenzyme in cells throughout the body; helps convert protein to energy.
- Helps to oxidize fatty acids.
- Aids in carbohydrate metabolism.
- Helps in the manufacture of growth hormones; adrenal hormone (ACTH); insulin; and thyroxine, a hormone required in metabolic processes.
- Helps control growth and development of the fetus; acts with vitamin E.

Symptoms of Deficiency
- Early symptoms include anxiety, loss of appetite, digestive problems and fatigue.
- Typical clinical symptoms of severe deficiency are cracks and fissures of the lips and corners of the mouth, fissures of the tongue and extreme redness of the tongue, greasy scaliness of the face around the nose and mouth, prominent new blood vessels in the whites of the eyes and a specific rash of the genital area in both men and women.
- Severe personality disorders due to interference with metabolism of nerve cells.

RDA

Infants: birth to 6 months	0.4 mg
6 months to 1 year	0.6 mg
Children: 1–3 years	0.8 mg
4–6 years	1.0 mg
7–10 years	1.4 mg
Males: 11–14 years	1.6 mg
15–22 years	1.7 mg
23–50 years	1.6 mg
51 years and over	1.4 mg

Females: 11–22 years	1.3 mg
23 years and over	1.2 mg
Pregnant women	an *extra* 0.3 mg
Lactating women	an *extra* 0.5 mg

Toxic Level
None reported even with ingestion of doses up to 5,000 times the recommended level.

Symptoms of Toxicity
None.

Vitamin B₃ (Niacin, Nicotinic Acid, Nicotinamide)

Sources
- *Animal sources of tryptophan*, capable of producing niacin (about 60 mg of tryptophan are required to produce 1 mg of niacin)—veal, beef, chicken, pork and lamb or mutton liver, as well as the meats themselves, fish, dairy products.
- *Plant sources of niacin*—whole-grain products, peanuts, yeast. (Coffee beans contain a form of niacin that is converted to usable niacin during roasting, so coffee drinkers may get a substantial amount of niacin from this source.) Some of the plant sources of this vitamin may be in metabolically unusable forms—some cereals, seeds, corn and certain vegetable greens.

Functions
- Acts as a coenzyme required for the metabolism of proteins, fats and carbohydrates.
- Helps maintain normal growth and energy supplies.
- Helps in the formation of bile salts needed to digest fats and absorb fat-soluble vitamins.
- Helps control formation of the hormones insulin, thyroxine and growth hormone.
- May help control blood levels of substances such as cholesterol and triglycerides that may contribute to cardiovascular disease.
- Helps in the functioning of the liver, skin, intestines and nervous system.

Symptoms of Deficiency
- Early symptoms are weakness, fatigue, poor appetite and indigestion, irritability, headache, memory loss.

- Classical symptoms of pellagra (common among poor people in the southern United States even today) include the 4 Ds—dermatitis (skin rash) on the exposed skin, which looks like sunburn in light-skinned people and areas of excessive darkness in darker-skinned people; diarrhea; dementia (psychosis); and eventual death.

RDA

Infants: birth to 6 months	6 mg
6 months to 1 year	8 mg
Children: 1–3 years	9 mg
4–6 years	11 mg
7–10 years	16 mg
Males: 11–18 years	18 mg
19–22 years	19 mg
23–50 years	18 mg
51 years and over	16 mg
Females: 11–14 years	15 mg
15–22 years	14 mg
23 years and over	13 mg
Pregnant women	an *extra* 2 mg
Lactating women	an *extra* 5 mg

Toxic Level
Generally regarded as nontoxic in levels under 3 grams to 4 grams daily.

Symptoms of Toxicity
- Large therapeutic doses (approximately 200 mg) usually cause flushing of the skin and sometimes itching when administered as nicotinic acid; nicotinamide is normally given because it does not cause this reaction.
- Prolonged high dosage is thought to cause some gastrointestinal irritation and perhaps liver damage.

Vitamin B₆ (Pyridoxine, Pyridoxal, Pyridoxamine)

Sources
- *Animal foods*—meats and beef, chicken and pork liver, fish (herring, salmon, mackerel, tuna).
- *Plant foods*—brewer's yeast, peanuts, molasses, spinach, soybeans, legumes, bananas, yams, walnuts, whole-grain products.

Functions

- Coenzyme for the manufacture of proteins from amino acids.
- Coenzyme for all cells—required for them to metabolize proteins and fats.
- Helps in the manufacture of fats from fatty acids in foods.
- More than 60 enzymes depend on B_6 in order to function.
- Controls formation and function of niacin.
- Required for proper formation or function of red blood cells, bile salts and many hormones needed for growth; formation of the skeleton; and reproductive functioning.
- Helps maintain the health of teeth and facial bones (as such, helps to prevent dental infections and cavities).
- A coenzyme in muscle, lymph, liver and nerve tissue.
- Helps in maintaining chemical balance in the tissues and helps regulate excretion of water.
- Aids in maintaining energy production and in resistance to stress.

Symptoms of Deficiency

- Prenatal deprivation results in mental retardation and blood disorders.
- Produces the sores of the skin, lips and tongue characteristic of B_2 and B_{12} deficiencies.
- Anemia and improper functioning of the white blood cells and disturbances in production of antibodies.
- Nervous system disorders include convulsions, abnormal brain waves, sleeplessness, confusion, nervousness, depression, irritability, interference with nerves that supply muscles and difficulties in movement of these muscles.

RDA

Infants: birth to 6 months	0.3 mg
6 months to 1 year	0.6 mg
Children: 1–3 years	0.9 mg
4–6 years	1.3 mg
7–10 years	1.6 mg
Males: 11–14 years	1.8 mg
15–18 years	2.0 mg
19 years and over	2.2 mg
Females: 11–14 years	1.8 mg
15 years and over	2.0 mg
Pregnant women	an *extra* 0.6 mg
Lactating women	an *extra* 0.5 mg

Toxic Level
One human study involving adults receiving 200 mg daily for 33 days showed increased subsequent requirements. Deficiency symptoms can result when normal doses are resumed following very large doses.

Symptoms of Toxicity
See "Toxic Level." Toxicity per se is only observed following doses as high as 1 gram per pound of body weight daily.

Vitamin B$_{12}$ (Cobalamin, Cyanocobalamin)

Sources
- Intestinal organisms.
- Liver; kidneys (pork, beef and lamb); egg yolks; fish, poultry and meats; milk and milk products.
- Plants contain no vitamin B$_{12}$ except for very tiny amounts in the nodules of the roots. *Vegetarians must take supplements if no eggs or dairy product are included in their diet.* Fermented soy and other oriental fermented foods (if available) can supply B$_{12}$.

Functions
- Acts as coenzyme in all cells and aids in the synthesis of important nucleic acids called DNA and RNA.
- Aids in the synthesis of proteins and fats from dietary intake.
- Essential to maintain the health of nerve cell tissues and tissue membranes.
- Important for bone marrow, the intestinal tract and the growth hormones.
- Acts as a coenzyme for metabolism in the liver, the kidney, the heart and nerve, bone and skin tissues.

Symptoms of Deficiency
- Early symptoms include memory loss, paranoia and exaggerated mood swings. These symptoms may be present for years before other symptoms are seen.
- Later symptoms are poor growth; poor carbohydrate metabolism; and degeneration of the nerves and spinal cord, which causes difficulties in walking, strange sensations in the skin, loss of reflexes, muscle spasticity.
- *Pernicious anemia* is the term used for persons whose symptoms occur as a result of atrophy of the stomach, a

condition in which there is no normal stomach acid and no special factor that is necessary for the utilization of vitamin B_{12}. This condition usually occurs in persons over 40 years of age and may be inherited.

RDA

Infants: birth to 6 months	0.5 μg
6 months to 1 year	1.5 μg
Children: 1–3 years	2.0 μg
4–6 years	2.5 μg
Males and females: 7 years and over	3.0 μg
Pregnant or lactating women	an *extra* 1.0 μg

Toxic Level
Not toxic even in large doses.

Symptoms of Toxicity
None known.

Folic Acid (Folacin, Folate)

Sources
- Intestinal bacteria manufacture small amounts.
- *Animal foods*—liver, kidney and heart of beef, lamb, pork and chicken; tuna.
- *Plant foods*—dark green leafy vegetables, legumes, nuts and whole grains, yeast.

Functions
- An essential coenzyme for all cells.
- Aids in the synthesis of DNA and RNA, choline and enzymes necessary for cell division.
- Regulates the development of nerve cells of the unborn.
- Is part of the genes of chromosomes of every cell.
- Helps maintain normal growth patterns.
- Helps maintain the nervous system, the intestinal tract, reproductive organs and white blood cells.
- Helps to construct amino acids.

Symptoms of Deficiency
- Weakness and weight loss.
- Cracking and redness of the tongue and mouth tissues.
- Diarrhea and poor digestion (inability to absorb certain food substances).

- Several forms of anemia (difficult to distinguish from those due to B_{12} deficiency).

RDA

Infants: birth to 6 months	30 μg
6 months to 1 year	45 μg
Children: 1–3 years	100 μg
4–6 years	200 μg
7–10 years	300 μg
Males and females: 11 years and over	400 μg
Pregnant women	an *extra* 400 μg
Lactating women	an *extra* 100 μg

Biotin (Vitamin H)

Sources
- Intestinal bacteria manufacture small amounts.
- Available in nearly all foods in small concentrations; particularly high in pork liver, salmon, chicken, yeast, wheat, corn and mushrooms.

Functions
- Important for fatty acid synthesis, as well as synthesis of proteins and carbohydrates in the body; aids in maintaining metabolism of these nutrients.
- Acts as a liver coenzyme in many types of metabolism.
- Aids in maintaining sweat glands, male sex glands, nerve tissue, bone marrow and the health of skin and hair.

Symptoms of Deficiency
No specific deficiency disease except that due to over-ingestion of raw egg whites, which inactivates biotin. This results in a set of symptoms known as "egg white injury"—cracked, red tongue; grayish mucous membranes; pale skin; depression; skin rash; painful and excessively sensitive skin (as the early symptoms). Later symptoms are lack of appetite, nausea, vomiting, anemia, high cholesterol levels in the blood.

RDA not established.
Figures represent safe and adequate daily intakes.

Infants: birth to 6 months	35 μg
6 months to 1 year	50 μg

Children: 1–3 years	65 µg
4–6 years	85 µg
7–10 years	120 µg
Males and females: 11 years and over (including pregnant and lactating women)	100–200 µg

Toxic Level
Not established.

Symptoms of Toxicity
Not seen.

Pantothenic Acid

Sources
- Found in all living things.
- *Best animal sources*—livers, egg yolks, herring, meats.
- *Best plant sources*—yeast, bran, raw peanuts, fresh vegetables, legumes.
- Oils, sugars and alcohol are nearly devoid of the vitamin.

Functions
- An essential coenzyme in the metabolism of carbohydrates, fats and proteins in all cells.
- Essential in the synthesis of nerve cell hormone (acetylcholine), growth hormone and adrenal hormones.
- Important for the formation of antibodies (prevention of infection).
- Required for the formation of body fats made from fatty acids.
- Promotes formation and normal functioning of amino acids.
- Aids in balancing amounts of tissue fluid.

Symptoms of Deficiency
- No specific deficiency disease.
- Early symptoms include loss of appetite, fatigue and constipation.
- Mental depression; physical weakness; disruption of nerve function, including strange sensations in hands and feet; sleeplessness. Personality changes and reduction in the formation of bile salts are seen later, along with increased susceptibility to infection.

RDA not established.
Figures represent safe and adequate daily intakes.

Infants: birth to 6 months	2 mg
6 months to 1 year	3 mg
Children: 1–3 years	3 mg
4–7 years	3–4 mg
7–10 years	4–5 mg
Males and females: 11 years and over	
(including pregnant and lactating women)	4–7 mg

Vitamin C (Ascorbic Acid)

Sources

- *Best sources*, contrary to popular opinion, are green peppers, parsley, broccoli, brussel sprouts, turnip greens and guava. Tomatoes, strawberries and citrus fruits are good but not the *best* sources. Green, leafy vegetables and even potatoes are relatively good sources.
- Milk (except for mother's milk) and meats are *poor* sources.

Functions

- An essential coenzyme in producing collagen (a structural protein), steroid hormones, pigment (coloring matter) and certain parts of cell and tissue membranes.
- Protects vitamins A and E from degradation by other substances.
- Regulates metabolism of amino acids.
- Important for strength of blood vessel walls, particularly the small vessels (capillaries).
- Protects membranes and tissues from injury from pollution, poisons and other substances.
- Promotes absorption of iron from foods.
- Helps wound healing; helps protect against the effects of stress; aids in regulating growth.
- Stimulates body defense against infection.
- Prevents conversion of food nitrites to nitrosamines (substances known to cause cancer).
- Helps in the formation of bones, teeth and cartilage.
- Helps in the production of adrenal and reproductive hormones.
- Aids in fat metabolism; may have some protective effect with regard to serum cholesterol levels.

Symptoms of Deficiency

Early signs are small hemorrhages into the skin, lethargy and tendency to infections. Gum infections and cavities are common, and there is swelling of the tissues throughout the body. Hair and skin become dry; the gums bleed; and teeth fall out. The eyes are dry, and hair falls out. There is joint pain and water in the joints, and the water in the tissues increases to a "pitting edema" (on pressing a finger into the legs, the mark or pit remains). Depression, hysteria and other emotional and mental symptoms may occur. Death can occur as symptoms grow increasingly worse. This set of symptoms is called scurvy and once was a common disease among sailors unable to get fresh vegetables and fruits as well as among many people in all parts of the world, rich and poor, with deficient diets.

RDA

Infants: birth to 1 year	35 mg
Children: 1–10 years	45 mg
11–14 years	50 mg
Males and females: 15 years and over	60 mg
Pregnant women	an *extra* 20 mg
Lactating women	an *extra* 40 mg

Toxic Level

Levels up to 1,000 mg daily are well tolerated; some people have taken up to 10 grams daily without toxic symptoms.

Symptoms of Toxicity (and/or Symptoms Noted with Large Intake)

- An increased incidence of uric acid and cystine stones in the urinary tract has been noted with people taking large doses of vitamin C. May cause false-positive results with urine diabetes tests.
- Vitamin C may cause large amounts of urine to be excreted.
- Digestive upsets are regarded by some as signs of toxicity, while others believe the symptoms are simple over-acidity. The diarrhea may be due to the vitamin C or to the filler substance used in vitamin supplements.
- Persons with some genetic disorders (glucose-6-phosphate dehydrogenase deficiency, which is common in black people) may suffer from vitamin B_{12} deficiency with high vitamin C levels.

Vitamin Supplements

In a perfect world, everyone would eat well-balanced meals and no one would need vitamin supplements. Of course, this is not the case. We are often hurried and turn to nutrient-poor "convenience" foods. We diet and limit our food (and nutrient) intake. We are picky eaters and fill up on our favorite foods while turning away from other foods that our bodies may require.

Many people do not get all the vitamins they need every day. The best remedy is to adjust our diet so that it supplies all vital nutrients. If a deficiency persists, a vitamin supplement may be called for. Consult your physician about what you may be lacking and how best to get it.

There are two ways to supplement vitamin intake: food itself or packaged supplements.

All vitamins are chemical substances, whether they occur naturally or are manufactured in laboratories. By taking the first choice, food, we are going to the source of the nutrients.

Packaged vitamin supplements, whether in the form of tablets, capsules, liquids or drops, have the advantage of coming in convenient, formulated doses. The bottles in which the vitamins are stored protect them from destructive heat, light and exposure to air. However, such protection is not infinite, and it is important to check the expiration date on the bottle prior to purchase. Keeping the bottle in a cool, dry, dark place will also help to maintain potency.

Bottled vitamins may be natural, that is, derived from specific foods, or they may be artificial. The body utilizes either form, despite the claims of some health-food advocates that natural vitamins are superior.

Vitamin capsules and pills are not suited to everyone. The nutrients are mixed with "filler" substances that have caused some people to experience digestive upsets. The law now requires manufacturers to list fillers on the bottle. Vitamin supplements vary widely in price. Since the most expensive are not necessarily the best, it is wise to compare brands and prices.

While supplements are valuable for compensating vitamin deficiencies, be aware that they cannot make up either for a basically poor and inadequate diet or for a generally unhealthy lifestyle.

Uses and Abuses of Vitamin Supplements

Although there is no unanimity of opinion about vitamin supplementation for the average person, certain individuals are generally conceded to require extra amounts of vitamins. The specific types of individuals and the reasons for their increased vitamin needs will be discussed below.

Alcoholics and "Heavy Drinkers"
Alcohol interferes with the absorption, utilization and storage of many vitamins, particularly those in the B group. Since vitamins are needed to metabolize alcohol and to repair the damage done by alcohol, requirements are necessarily increased. In addition, many heavy drinkers obtain much of their caloric intake from the alcohol itself, thereby leading to a poor intake of nutrients in general. Supplementation is generally required.

Pregnant and Nursing Women
Vitamin and mineral supplementation is commonly prescribed for pregnant and nursing women, who, in different ways, need additional nourishment. Normally, the woman's increased caloric intake should meet her increased need for nutrients of all kinds, but this is often not the case, and it is better to err on the side of plenty. Morning sickness, food cravings and inability to tolerate certain foods can make the need for supplementation more imperative. Since fetal needs are not always coincident with maternal intake, and since the developing fetus is more vulnerable to both deprivation and excess, all supplementation should be under medical guidance.

Heavy Smokers
Persons smoking a pack of cigarettes daily require about 40 percent more vitamin C than other individuals. It has been estimated that they require about 100 mg daily in excess of normal requirements. This can be made up by eating vitamin-rich foods or by taking a vitamin supplement.

Persons Under Stress
All forms of stress—illness, surgery, burns, even psychological stress—can deplete the body reserves and cause increased need for vitamins, especially vitamin C. In addition, particular types of illness are associated with difficulties in absorption of certain nutrients. Chronic intestinal disorders are associated with deficiencies in the fat-soluble vitamins. Other intestinal diseases may interfere with the absorption of the water-soluble B vitamins, particularly vitamin B_{12}. Specific states will be mentioned in the sections devoted to each vitamin.

Elderly People

Food absorption and metabolism are common problems in elderly people, and in many the amount and type of food intake further complicates the matter. The B vitamins and C are particularly likely to be poorly absorbed. Many elderly people could benefit from daily mineral and vitamin supplementation.

Persons on Weight-Reduction Diets

People who wish to lose weight, particularly a large amount of weight, may need to be on diets for relatively long periods of time and *may* need vitamin supplements. This is especially true of individuals who are fasting or are attempting to lose a great deal of weight in a short period of time. However, if a diet is balanced and weight loss is gradual, there may be no need for supplements. Generally, women on a diet of less than 1,200 calories a day need supplements.

People who are on restricted diets for any reason are more likely to require vitamin and mineral supplements. If the diet is restricted for medical reasons, the physician will probably prescribe supplementation at the same time as the diet.

Persons Receiving Certain Medications—Drug and Vitamin Interactions

Perhaps the most widely prescribed medications requiring vitamin supplementation are the oral contraceptives. The B vitamins, particularly B_6, and vitamin C appear to be those most frequently affected by the metabolic changes caused by birth control pills.

Long-term antibiotic therapy can destroy certain intestinal bacteria that produce some of the B vitamins and vitamin K. Folacin deficiency can result from drugs used to treat epilepsy, some drugs used to treat cancer and drugs used to treat malaria. Some oral anti-diabetic drugs can interfere with the absorption of vitamin B_{12}. One of the anti-tuberculosis drugs, INH, can produce deficiencies of both niacin and vitamin B_6. Some diuretics (water pills) and penicillamine (used to treat severe arthritis) can also cause B_6 deficiency. The use of antacids can destroy vitamin C, and laxative usage can markedly interfere with the absorption of a wide variety of vitamins. Prolonged aspirin usage has been known to interfere with vitamin B_{12} absorption, can destroy vitamin C and may cause a deficiency in vitamin K.

Not only can drugs interfere with vitamins, but large doses of vitamins can interfere with drug therapy. For example, vitamin C in large doses can magnify the effects of oral anti-diabetic drugs and can confuse the results of tests for sugar in the urine by giving a false-positive result. Certain B vitamins and vitamin E can alter the patient's response to anticoagulant drugs (those that prevent blood clotting) and some drugs used to lower blood pressure.

Obviously, if you are under care for any medical condition, or are receiving any drugs and are planning to take vitamin supplements, you should consult your physician. In addition, if your blood, urine or other body fluids are to be tested, your doctor and the person performing the test should be informed of your additional vitamin intake.

Table 7.1 details some of the known effects of vitamin interactions with drugs and other substances. Although these are by no means all of the possible interactions, they do point up the importance of checking to make certain of possible interactions between any medications, including those you buy without prescription, and other substances you might use or that might be present in your foods and the vitamins you require—in whatever form you take them. It is wise to check with your doctor and your druggist about any possible interactions.

TABLE 7.1
VITAMIN INTERACTIONS WITH DRUGS AND OTHER SUBSTANCES

Antacids	Interfere with vitamin C
Antibiotics	Interfere with most of the vitamin B group and vitamin K
Anticoagulants	Vitamin E alters patient's response; interfere with vitamins C and K
Anticonvulsants	Interfere with vitamin D
Antidepressants	Interfere with vitamin C
Anti-diabetic agents (oral)	Vitamin C can magnify their effects; they may interfere with vitamin B_{12}
Antihypertensives	Vitamin E can alter patient's response
Aspirin and aspirin substitutes	Interfere with vitamins K, B_{12}, C
Baking soda	Interferes with vitamin B_1
Chloramphenicol	Interferes with vitamin B_{12}
Codeine	Interferes with vitamin B_{12}
Contraceptives (oral)	Interfere with vitamins C, E, B_1, B_2, B_6, B_{12}, folic acid
Cortisone and prednisone	Interfere with vitamin C, vitamin B_6, vitamin D

Diuretics	Interfere with vitamin C
Hydralazine	Interferes with vitamin B_6
Indomethacin	Interferes with vitamin C
Iron	Interferes with vitamin E when taken with iron; vitamin C enhances iron absorption
Isoniazid (INH)	Interferes with vitamin B_6
Methotrexate	Interferes with folic acid
Methylbromide (preservative)	Interferes with pantothenic acid
Mineral oil	Interferes with fat-soluble vitamins A, E, K
Neomycin	Interferes with vitamin B_{12}
Penicillamine	Interferes with vitamin B_6
"Rancid" fats and oils. Fats and oils are used both as foods and as carriers for medicines. If old and "rancid," they can	Interfere with vitamin E
Steroids (hormones)	Interfere with vitamin C
Thyroid hormones	Interfere with vitamin E

Megadoses

Some of us may have a friend who pops a couple of 500 mg tablet of rose hips (vitamin C) every day and confidently boasts that h or she hasn't had a cold in three years.

Such people may not have caught a cold recently, but the have been captured by one of the most prevalent myths associate with vitamins. Research to date has found *no* evidence tha vitamin C prevents the common cold, although there is som evidence that the vitamin might help lessen the severity of som symptoms of the ailment. Unless otherwise advised by a physi cian, an adult needs no more than the RDA, 60 mg, of vitamin C

Those who swear by vitamin C, whether they know it or no are part of the megadosing fad. The fad involves taking vitami doses far in excess of the RDAs in the belief that extraordinar medical benefits will result. If the faddists are to be believe megadoses of vitamins will do everything from relieving unde arm odor to curing cancer. Dozens of books and magazine article appear every year touting this or that vitamin as the latest "miracle cure" and urging readers to increase their vitamin intakes drastically.

The advocates of megadosing base their claims on simple logic: If a little of a good thing is good for you, then a lot of a good thing must be great for you. This logic, however, does not necessarily hold true when applied to vitamins.

For example, it is known that vitamin A is good for the eyes. However, it cannot be concluded that any problem with vision can be corrected by megadoses of vitamin A. In a similar manner, problems affecting other portions of the body or other functions cannot be corrected by taking vitamins unless the original problem was vitamin-related.

It is helpful to remember the nature of vitamin storage in the body. Fat-soluble vitamins (A, D, E and K) can be stored in large quantities sufficient to last for months. Water-soluble vitamins (B and C), once they reach a certain level in the body, are readily excreted in urine and perspiration.

Therefore, megadoses of fat-soluble vitamins are usually unnecessary, and they can be toxic. (An overdose of vitamin A in particular can have serious medical consequences.) And while there is far less danger of reaching a toxic level with water-soluble vitamins, megadoses may at best be useless.

Of course, it should be mentioned that not everyone has the same vitamin requirements, nor have requirements been established for all vitamins. Government authorities freely admit that the RDAs are estimates based on the clinical observation of test groups. Also, certain people (for example, pregnant women) may need vitamins in doses above the RDAs.

These considerations lead to the conclusion that it is best to consult a physician before taking vitamin supplements or joining the megadosing fad. With vitamins, as with other essential nutrients, it *is* possible to have too much of a good thing.

Facts Versus Fads

As recently as 1940, only 10 of the 13 vitamins we have discussed had been identified. Today, the manufacture of vitamin supplements is a lucrative business.

It would be comforting to think that every person buying those products is doing so merely to make up for some minor vitamin deficiencies in his or her daily diet. But we know otherwise. Thousands of people are wasting their money, and perhaps endangering their health, by taking vitamins they don't need.

True, we have individualized vitamin requirements. And it is just as true that we would like to believe that swallowing a fistful of vitamins regularly will cure our ills, heighten or restore our sexual potency or slow the aging process.

Vitamins are not medicine, and they will not perform miracles. No one should attempt to treat a possible or actual illness with self-styled vitamin therapy. And no one should rely on vitamins to prevent illness—no matter what our friends tell us about vitamin C. The best way of making sure you get the vitamins you need to keep you healthy is to eat a balanced diet.

Chapter 8

Minerals

Minerals are inorganic substances, which means they are not formed by living matter and contain no carbon. All organic material contains carbon and once was part of, or was produced by, living plants or animals. Our continuing need for minerals in our diet, even though in the most tiny quantities, in many instances reflects our link with our ancient heritage of the sea. The major salts from seawater in various combinations are the same as the salts in our cells and body fluids. Their names are familiar—sodium, potassium, calcium and magnesium—as are the combinations with chloride, phosphate and carbonate. The most common combination is sodium chloride, or ordinary table salt, which is discussed in a separate chapter.

We will discuss the most common major minerals required by the body as well as the identified trace elements (those appearing in very minute quantities in the body). We say "identified" because, as with the vitamins, more is learned about essential requirements as studies continue. Some minerals are present in the body in such tiny amounts that until recently they had not been identified, nor is much known about their activity in the body. One fact is known about all the minerals, however: They work together, as do many of the vitamins. In the delicate balance of body functioning, each vital substance plays its own special part; too much of a substance throws the whole balance off, and when the balance is askew, symptoms appear to tell us that something is wrong. Slowly we are becoming wise enough to interpret some of these symptoms and help the body return to normal functioning. The roles of the minerals, our current understanding of what affects these roles and the foods that enable the body to obtain sufficient amounts will be discussed. Factors that help in absorption and utilization of the minerals, as well as those that interfere, will also be presented, as will the ailments that can occur when vital mineral balance is compromised. Interactions and needs for supplements appear only where appropriate. RDAs are provided where they have been established; in other cases, only government estimates, "Estimated Safe and Adequate Daily Intake," are given because that is the only information currently available.

In general, the minerals function in the body in four roles:

1. As cofactors in various metabolic reactions.
2. As part of compounds that contain organic matter (enzymes, vitamins, hormones, certain elements in the blood).
3. As electrically charged elements (ions) important in making possible the movement of substances across body cell membranes and the movements of muscles.
4. As elements in bone structure.

Although minerals are of vital importance, they make up only about 4 percent of the body's weight; all of the trace minerals account for only about .01 percent of total body weight.

The Major Minerals in the Body

The major minerals are so designated on the basis of the amounts required in the diet, not on their relative importance. The major minerals are also called "macrominerals." These are calcium, phosphorus, magnesium, potassium, sulfur, chloride and sodium (the last of which will be discussed in a separate chapter, as mentioned).

Calcium

Calcium is the most abundant mineral in the body, accounting for about 2 percent of body weight. This amounts to approximately 1,250 grams, of which 99 percent is in the bones and teeth. About 1 percent is in the soft tissues, where it is necessary for blood clotting, for the proper functioning of muscles and nerve tissue (so-called excitability), the contractility of muscles and the normal functioning of the special muscle in the walls of the heart. Calcium is also a vital cofactor in the manufacture of certain enzymes.

Only about 1 percent of body calcium is in the teeth, the remaining 98 percent not required for metabolic function being in the bones. Although these areas are vital, as far as the body's needs are concerned, the 1 percent required for metabolic function comes first; and if necessary, the body will deplete calcium from bones and teeth to meet its more vital calcium needs.

RDA*

Infants: up to 6 months	360 mg
6 months to 1 year	540 mg
Children: 1–10 years	800 mg
Males and females: 11–18 years	1,200 mg
19 years and over	800 mg
Pregnant and nursing women	an *extra* 400 mg

*See footnote on p. 116 for information about the reliability of these RDA figures.

Effects of Calcium Deficiency

Because of the body's tendency to rob bones and teeth of calcium to supply other needs, it has been suggested that 800 mg of calcium daily, particularly for adult women, may not be sufficient. Many physicians recommend 1,000 mg daily for premenopausal women and up to 1,500 mg daily postmenopausally. Let us take a look at the reasoning behind this.

It has been found that the body first robs from the jawbone, which may account for the prevalence of periodontal disease among adults, particularly women. Years ago, women used to claim that they would lose a tooth for each child. Since the needs of the fetus come first, as we have also discovered with other nutrients, if the diet is deficient in calcium, the fetus gets first claim. As you know, in periodontal disease, the tooth itself may be sound, and yet the bone around the tooth "demineralizes"; the socket fails to hold the tooth any longer; and so the tooth falls out. This is also common in older persons in general, many of whom have a long-standing calcium deficiency.

So-called dowager's hump is also reflective of calcium deficiency (among other things), as is osteoporosis, or thinning of the bones throughout the body. The fact that old people are shorter than when they were young is not simply because they *don't* stand straight; it is often because they *cannot* stand straight, since the bones have literally squashed together in the spine, due both to numerous fractures in the vertebrae (spine segments) and to thinning of the "padding" between these bony segments. The fractures occur because of lack of calcium, which has made the bones fragile and subject to fracture. In children the lack of calcium results in the disease called "rickets." The children typically have bowed legs and retarded growth. In many instances the "calcium" deficiency is not so much a deficiency of calcium as it is a deficiency of vitamin D, which interacts with calcium (as discussed below) and is required for good development and maintenance of bones and teeth. We will later examine other factors that affect calcium usage.

Let us look at other situations in which the body shows evidence of calcium deficiency. One thing that will demineralize the bones very effectively is lack of activity, which is one reason why exercise is so valuable throughout life. It is also a major reason why activity is encouraged as soon as possible after any injury or surgery. The "weakness" that occurs with bed rest is partly due to the demineralization of the bones. Even if a perfectly healthy person went to bed and stayed there for even several days, the same thing would happen. Not only would the bones lose the minerals but the minerals would be diverted to the urinary tract in large amounts. This is another reason why people who are in bed a lot or for a prolonged time develop "stones" in the kidneys. So activity is truly a medicine in its own right, both preventively and therapeutically.

One rather rugged group of people who are also prone to develop these problems is the astronauts. Space flight or weight-lessness encourages bone loss even after a few days in space. And it encourages excessive loss of minerals in the urine. The problem is for scientists to find ways for astronauts to exercise while in space to prevent this from happening. It is weight bearing that is the problem, not just movement per se.

Calcium Interactions

In order for calcium to be properly absorbed and used in the body, other important substances are required. One of them is vitamin D, which regulates the absorption of calcium and phosphorus from the intestinal tract. Calcium, phosphorus and magnesium work together for normal growth and maintenance of bony structures. Perhaps you tend to think of bones as static dead things, except during periods of growth in childhood and adolescence. But this is not so. Our bones replace about $1/5$ of their total calcium each year, and there is a constant movement of calcium in and out of the bones both for repair and to maintain a constant level of calcium in the blood and other body fluids.

Calcium is needed for the proper absorption and utilization of vitamin B_{12} and, in conjunction with vitamin B_6, is important in burning proteins when they are required for energy. As a matter of fact, whenever high protein consumption occurs for any reason (it is often necessary for persons with hypoglycemia), the body has extra needs for calcium. And, whenever there is a need for extra calcium, there is also a need for added zinc, because calcium decreases the absorption of zinc. The interaction between vitamin D and calcium is clearly shown in normal growth and development of bones and teeth and also in the fact that the often dangerously low levels of calcium in persons with kidney disease may be due to their inability to metabolize vitamin D and transform it into a biologically useful form.

It is thought that calcium in the water supply (one of the minerals that make water "hard") can help to prevent absorption of lead and cadmium in the pipes or soil that can lead to toxicity. Another interesting interaction involving calcium is its relationship to lithium, a chemical used in treating depression. One authority has noted that lithium lowers the level of calcium in the blood and leads to retention of calcium elsewhere in the body. If this shift in calcium metabolism does not take place, it is unlikely that the patient will respond to lithium treatment.

Effects of Excessive Calcium
Too much calcium can prevent coagulation of the blood and also result in retarded growth and digestive upsets in children. In addition, high levels can interfere with the absorption of zinc, iron and manganese as well as causing undue fatigue. The buildup of calcium in the tissues and the kidneys may be due as much to low levels of magnesium and vitamin B_6 as to high levels of calcium.

Meeting Calcium Needs
Table 8.1 lists a number of calcium-rich foods. It is wise to note, however, that certain foods interfere with proper absorption of calcium or increase calcium loss:

- Soft drinks—because they contain excessive amounts of phosphorus.
- High-fat or high-protein diets.
- Excessive amounts of spinach, rhubarb, swiss chard, beet greens and bran—because they contain oxalic acid or phytic acid, which prevents absorption.

Calcium Supplements
It is difficult to take calcium supplements in large amounts because the pills are *huge*, but since calcium needs continue throughout life, dry milk powders can be used in food preparation as well as hard cheeses for those who do not drink or cannot drink

TABLE 8.1
CALCIUM IN SELECTED FOODS

Food	Quantity	Milligrams
Almonds, shelled	1 cup	304
Beet greens, cooked	1 cup	144
Broccoli, cooked	1 stalk	158
Cabbage, white mustard, cooked	1 cup	252
Cashew nuts, roasted in oil	1 cup	150
Cheese, cheddar	1 oz.	204
Cheese, cottage, low fat (2%)	1 cup	155
Cheese, Parmesan, grated	1 oz.	390
Cheese, ricotta, part skim milk	1 cup	669
Cheese, Swiss	1 oz.	219
Collards, cooked	1 cup	357
Cream, sour	1 cup	268
Cream, sweet, half-and-half (cream and milk)	1 cup	254
Cream, sweet, heavy (unwhipped)	1 cup	154
Custard, baked	1 cup	297
Farina, enriched	1 cup	147
Filberts (hazelnuts), chopped	1 cup	240
Ice cream, hard	1 cup	176
Kale, cooked (without stems and ribs)	1 cup	206
Milk, chocolate (commercial), low fat (1%)	1 cup	287
Milk, low fat (1%), no milk solids added	1 cup	300
Milk, malted, chocolate (1 cup whole milk with 3 tsp. malted milk powder)	1 cup	304
Milk, malted, natural	1 cup	347
Milk, skim, no milk solids added	1 cup	302
Milk, whole (3.3% fat)	1 cup	291
Oysters, raw	1 cup	226
Peanuts, salted, roasted in oil	1 cup	107
Pudding, chocolate (from mix)	1 cup	265

TABLE 8.1
CALCIUM IN SELECTED FOODS

Food	Quantity	Milligrams
Pudding, vanilla (from home recipe)	1 cup	298
Rhubarb, cooked, sugar added	1 cup	211
Salmon, pink, canned	3 oz.	243
Sardines, canned in oil	3 oz.	424
Spinach, cooked	1 cup	167
Yogurt, made with nonfat milk	1 cup	452

SOURCE: Adapted from L. Patrick Coyle, *The World Encyclopedia of Food* (New York: Facts On File, 1982), pp. 432–475.

milk. For those with milk allergy or lack of lactase (an enzyme required to help in proper digestion of milk), drinking acidophilus milk or putting lactase in milk can solve the problem. On the other hand, yogurt serves the same purpose, and there is no problem in terms of lactase. Buttermilk, sour cream and other forms that have prior bacterial activity likewise are acceptable to people with low lactase levels.

Phosphorus

The body maintains an almost constant 1.5 to 1 ratio of calcium to phosphorus, a ratio that is vital in order to promote proper bone growth and maintenance. About 80 percent of phosphorus is in the bones and teeth. The remaining 20 percent has a number of functions. It helps to form the phospholipids, some carbohydrates, the nucleoproteins, vitamin B_6 and thiamine, and uncounted other organic compounds. One of the most important functions of phosphorus is in the formation of the special energy compounds ATP, GTP and UDP, which in a very complex fashion are involved in the derivation of energy from fats, carbohydrates and proteins and also in the storage of energy.

Like calcium, phosphorus is intimately involved with vitamin D and with two hormones, calcitonin and parathyroid hormone, in their metabolism at three sites—the intestine, the bones and the kidneys.

RDA*

Infants: up to 6 months	240 mg
6 months to 1 year	360 mg
Children: 1–10 years	800 mg
Males and females: 11–18 years	1,200 mg
19 years and over	800 mg
Pregnant and nursing women	an *extra* 400 mg

*These RDAs are somewhat unrealistic, as are those shown earlier for calcium, since the data on which they are based are considered somewhat unreliable. Since we know that blood levels of phosphorus in normal adults range from 3.0 to 4.0 mg per 100 ml and those for calcium are about 10 mg per 100 ml, it is obvious that the RDAs should not be the same.

The 1.5 to 1 calcium to phosphorus ratio—the ratio on which the RDAs were loosely based—was derived from a midpoint between the ratios found in cow's milk (1.2 to 1) and breast milk (2 to 1). It was felt that this ratio would prevent hypocalcemic (low-calcium) tetany (sharp flexion of the wrists and ankle joints, cramps in the muscles and convulsions) in newborns—a condition caused by excessive amounts of phosphorus. Children do, however, require more phosphorus for cell metabolism and growth. Their phosphorus levels in the blood are from 4.0 to 6.0 mg per 100 ml. The diet of the average American is far more likely to have an overabundance of phosphorus than calcium, and this should be taken into account when planning a diet.

Effects of Phosphorus Deficiency
Weakness, loss of appetite, malaise and bone pain can result from a lack of phosphorus. (As mentioned, however, the lack of phosphorus is unlikely.) In general, the symptoms are similar to those associated with calcium deficiency.

Phosphorus Interactions
As mentioned, phosphorus acts in concert with calcium, vitamin D and magnesium for processes affecting bone growth and maintenance. Adequate vitamin C prevents deposition of calcium and phosphorus when there is an oversupply of vitamin D. Excessive absorption of calcium indicates hyper-reactivity to vitamin D. Too much phosphorus can interfere with proper metabolism of calcium and can cause hypocalcemic tetany in children, as mentioned. Tetany can also result from insufficient vitamin D, which results in abnormal calcium and phosphorus metabolism.

Meeting Phosphorus Needs
Since calcium and phosphorus are so interdependent, it is best to meet the needs for both from the same foods and avoid the high phosphorus present in some processed foods and soft drinks. Milk and milk products, eggs, fish, dried beans and peas contain good quantities of both. Meat and poultry are also high in phosphorus (but not in calcium).

Phytic acid, which can interfere with the absorption of many trace minerals, is a phosphate and accounts for about 86 percent of the phosphorus in seeds. This source is bound, however, so that the sprouted seeds are a better source of phosphorus and also a better source of inositol, one of the vitamin B group considered to be involved in fat metabolism and called by some "the sleep vitamin."

Magnesium
Magnesium is involved in many of the same metabolic processes as are phosphorus and calcium. Therefore, it is not surprising to

find that magnesium is important in the building of bones and teeth, for the manufacture of proteins and DNA, for the production and transfer of energy, for muscle contraction, for normal nerve function (excitability) and as a cofactor in the production of many enzymes. It also aids in the body's adjustment to cold. Although it is an essential constituent of all soft tissue, 55 percent to 70 percent of the magnesium is found in the bones.

Magnesium is not only essential for normal calcium and phosphorus metabolism but is an important factor in keeping blood levels of cholesterol lowered. In this role it is considered protective against atherosclerosis. As an element in "hard" water, it is considered preventive in many forms of cardiovascular disease, although the exact mechanism is not known. Perhaps some of its protective ability may have to do with its ability to lower blood pressure. It is often used in this fashion for women who have toxemia of pregnancy. It is also required for glucose metabolism and hence is an ingredient in solutions given intravenously. There is also evidence that magnesium may be helpful in the treatment of some behavior disorders. This may not be too surprising since, along with zinc, magnesium is the mineral in highest concentration in the area of the brain called the "hippocampus," which is part of the "limbic system" known to be involved with emotions and behavior. Patients on lithium (an antidepressant) have been shown to have high blood levels of magnesium and calcium.

Magnesium is of value as a cathartic (epsom salts and milk of magnesia) and can deaden hunger (though this is not a recommended usage: Beware dieters—excessive diarrhea can result).

RDA

Infants: up to 6 months	50 mg
6 months to 1 year	70 mg
Children: 1–3 years	150 mg
4–6 years	200 mg
7–10 years	250 mg
Males: 11–14 years	350 mg
15–18 years	400 mg
19 years and over	350 mg
Females: 11 years and over	300 mg
Pregnant and nursing women	an *extra* 150 mg

Effects of Magnesium Deficiency

As mentioned, low levels of magnesium can cause both abnormal deposits of calcium in various tissues and kidney stones, as well as muscular twitching and tremors, irregular heartbeat, difficulty in sleeping, cramps in legs and feet, and shaky hands (similar to those of calcium and phosphorus deficiency). Persons with prolonged diarrhea, kidney disease, epilepsy or alcoholism, or those who take diuretics, are prone to magnesium deficiency. Persons with arteriosclerosis are likely to have low magnesium levels.

Because processing of grains and sugar destroys magnesium, as do water-softening agents and boiling of vegetables, relative deficiencies may be more common than supposed, even though magnesium sources are abundant in nature. Severe deficiency is less likely; it is marked by confusion, depression, disorientation and hallucinations (even delirium tremens). The possibility of this occurring in alcoholics is greater than with most other people, although severely ill people who are unable to eat for a period of time and whose magnesium is not restored through intravenous feedings might have this pattern of symptoms.

Magnesium Interactions

In the sulfate forms, magnesium cannot be absorbed; hence, it has laxative properties. Chemical fertilizers reduce the magnesium content of plants because they inhibit absorption of magnesium from the soil and the plants.

Effects of Excessive Magnesium

Magnesium toxicity is very rare, occurring only in conditions where there is insufficient urination or there is greatly increased absorption. Sometimes this can happen after an injection of magnesium. Women with certain types of cancer or patients with bone tumors can have an excess of magnesium. Since magnesium is sometimes used as an anesthetic agent, symptoms of toxicity are the same as with any other anesthesia excess—disturbed central nervous system functioning and possible death. In normal, healthy people, excess of magnesium is unknown.

Meeting Magnesium Needs

Whole-grain products, nuts and seeds, and green leafy vegetables (eaten raw) are the best sources of magnesium. Seafood is variable in its magnesium content, but can be good.

Magnesium Supplements

Because magnesium occurs generally in foods, particularly vegetables, a dietary deficiency appears to be rare among Americans with balanced diets. It is generally seen in pathological conditions such as chronic malabsorption syndrome, chronic renal failure and chronic alcoholism. There may be some advantages in the combination of magnesium and calcium (see "Calcium Interactions") available in dolomite, a naturally occurring combination of these minerals. The use of bone meal is questionable as a source of any mineral because calcium often serves to remove toxic chemicals from the body and naturally does so for all animals. Hence, bones may be filled with lead and other toxic materials.

Potassium

Along with sodium, chloride and bicarbonate, potassium is classed as a major electrolyte (a substance carrying electrical charges) with the vital task of controlling fluid balance in the cells and tissues throughout the body. It is also involved in muscle contraction, the transmission of nerve impulses, and the release of energy from carbohydrates, fats and proteins. Because of its action on muscles and as an electrolyte, potassium is particularly important in maintaining proper heart rhythm.

In addition, potassium may have some role in cholesterol metabolism and is reputedly helpful in relieving migraine headaches. In conjunction with phosphorus, potassium is vital in carrying oxygen to the brain cells.

The Food and Nutrition Board of the National Academy of Sciences—National Research Council recommended the following daily intake levels of potassium for healthy persons. Lack of adequate data prevented the board from establishing more precise amounts.

Estimated Safe and Adequate Daily Intake

Infants: up to 6 months	350–925 mg
6 months to 1 year	425–1,275 mg
Children: 1–3 years	550–1,650 mg
4–6 years	775–2,325 mg
7–10 years	1,000–3,000 mg
Children and adolescents: 11 years and over	1,525–4,575 mg
Adults	1,875–5,625 mg

Effects of Potassium Deficiency

The pronounced weakening of the muscles with lack of potassium is seen most importantly in the heart muscle. Heart attacks are frequently associated with low potassium levels. Low blood sugar, hypoglycemia, is also seen with potassium deficiency. Indigestion and intestinal gas due to weakness of intestinal muscle walls is also experienced, as well as retention of water in the tissues (edema).

People who take diuretics, those who are taking cortisone or ACTH, those who are taking digitalis or those who have diabetes, high blood pressure or liver disease need extra potassium, and if they do not get it, they may show symptoms of deficiency. These are abnormal heart rhythm, weakness and lethargy, and even failure of the lung and kidney function. People who work in intense heat and those who take laxatives or have prolonged diarrhea may develop some of these symptoms.

Potassium Interactions
Since potassium metabolism and deficiency are related so closely to those of sodium, *it is important to read the chapter on salt* (sodium chloride).

Effects of Excessive Potassium
Too much potassium can cause abnormalities of heart rhythm as well as weakness of the muscles and paralysis. It is important to realize that some of the symptoms of deficiency are similar to those of excess. The chance of excessive potassium intake is very slim, however, and usually results from an unintentional overdosage of oral or intravenous potassium. One must be careful of potassium supplements.

Meeting Potassium Needs
Green leafy vegetables, wheat germ, citrus juices, beans, lentils, bananas, nuts, dried dates, prunes and all fruits are good potassium sources, as are coffee, tea and cocoa.

Potassium Supplements
Potassium supplements may be required, particularly for people on diuretics (water pills). Unfortunately, the tablet supplements often upset the stomach, and the coated tablets can cause ulcers in the small intestine. Extra intake of potassium-rich foods may be preferred if enough can be eaten to make up the deficit. Otherwise, follow your physician's recommendations and report any symptoms promptly. Sometimes one type of supplement may suit one person but not another.

It is also important to remember that during cooking, the potassium may be leached out of many vegetables containing potassium. If the cooking water is then used in other cooking or in juices, that much potassium becomes available.

Sulfur

Sulfur, an important nutrient, is part of every cell as a component of sulfur-containing amino acids. It helps to form nails, hair and skin. Joints are also high in sulfur. It is interesting to note that curly hair depends on sulfur. Lotions to straighten hair and those to curl it can dissolve the hair if it is too fine. Like potassium, sulfur is inside the cells rather than outside as sodium is. It is thought that sulfur may act as a cofactor with taurine (an amino acid) in helping control membrane excitability in epilepsy and perhaps inhibit the biochemical changes in aging. Sulfur has been used successfully in the treatment of psoriasis, and it is thought that it may have value in other disorders of the nails and skin.

Sulfur is also a part of the thiamine and biotin structures (members of the vitamin B complex). One of the most obvious things about sulfur is its smell—terrible. It is one of the ways in which we recognize rotten eggs. The sulfur smell is present to some degree in fresh eggs also. And garlic and onions—those pervasive odors and the gas that provokes tears are a contribution of sulfur. Folklore attributes many healing qualities to these smelly but delicious plants, and perhaps this is right. They can lower blood pressure. Sulfur can also normalize bacteria in the intestinal tract when they are disturbed in quantity and metabolism due to antibiotic therapy. Sulfates are laxatives, too. Since sulfur occurs in the soil as a water-soluble salt, it can be depleted, as can other minerals (iodine, zinc, selenium), making any plants grown in such soil deficient in these important trace elements.

Sulfur-containing amino acids are protective against pollutants, and sulfur has been used with some success in helping to treat behavioral problems in children. No RDAs have yet been established, although one authority suggests adults need about 800 mg daily.

Effects of Sulfur Deficiency or Excess

Little is known about either lack or overdosage of sulfur at the present time. The general recommendation regarding intake for sheep is 0.2 percent of elemental sulfur (sheep and other ruminants change the sulfate to sulfur in the body). It is thought that persons with joint problems such as rheumatism and arthritis could benefit from sulfur, but there are no commercially available dietary supplements containing sulfur.

Meeting Sulfur Needs

Most dietary needs are met through the sulfur-containing amino acids—cysteine, cystine and methionine (the first two can be made from methionine in the body). Vegetarians can obtain sulfur from eggs, but if they do not eat eggs, a druggist will (upon request from a physician) fill capsules with sulfur flowers. The best dietary sources are protein foods from animal sources, wheat germ, brussels sprouts, lentils, onions, hot peppers, and of course, *garlic*.

Chloride

Like sodium, potassium and bicarbonate, chloride is one of the electrolytes (carrying electrical charges). These electrolytes are important in fluid balance and movement of substances across cell membranes. Chloride stimulates gastric juices (hydrochloric acid and other stomach digestive juices) and helps to remove waste from the body. It also aids in the distribution of hormones.

Estimated Safe and Adequate Daily Intake

Infants: up to 6 months	275–700 mg
6 months to 1 year	400–1,200 mg
Children: 1–3 years	500–1,500 mg
4–6 years	700–2,100 mg
7–10 years	925–2,775 mg
Children and adolescents: 11 years and over	1,400–4,200 mg
Adults	1,700–5,100 mg

Effects of Chloride Deficiency
Chloride deficiency is rather rare, since—when combined in sodium chloride as regular table salt (see separate chapter on salt)—it is overabundant in the diet. However, people taking diuretics, those with excessive fluid loss (diarrhea, vomiting, severe burns, fever), certain diseases causing excessive water intake (which means excessive dilution of the electrolytes and increased urination) or persons over-treated with intravenous fluids can develop both fluid and electrolyte loss and/or imbalance.

Effects of Excessive Chloride
Obviously an excess of chloride (usually in the form of salt) can cause a disturbance of fluid/electrolyte balance. There is a tendency to hold more water in the tissues when excessive sodium chloride is present—a problem that will be further discussed in the chapter on salt.

Meeting Chloride Needs
In addition to the chloride contained in salt, green leafy vegetables, raw meats, beets and radishes are good sources of chloride.

The Trace Minerals in the Body

Trace minerals are found in the body only in very small quantities. In fact, the quantities are so tiny that they comprise only .01 percent of the body's total weight. Scientists do not yet know how many trace minerals are essential for good nutrition. Among those considered important by the federal government are iron, zinc, iodine, copper, manganese, fluoride, chromium, selenium and molybdenum.

Iron

Iron is probably the best-known of the mineral elements, partly because there has been more advertising about "iron in the blood," which children equate with "Popeye and spinach" and their elders with "Geritol." The most important function of iron is to combine with protein to form hemoglobin, the oxygen-carrying component of the blood. Eighty-five percent of the total body iron is used in this fashion, with 5 percent found in muscle protein and a small amount within the cells. A portion of the brain also contains a high percentage of iron. All of these compounds are vital for cell respiration, in which oxygen and carbon dioxide are exchanged. The rest of the iron in the body is used in certain enzymes. Iron can be stored temporarily in a soluble plasma protein or in an insoluble form in the liver. It is this form that is important when considering iron overload, which will be discussed later.

RDA

Infants: up to 6 months	10 mg
6 months to 1 year	15 mg
Children: 1–3 years	15 mg
4–10 years	10 mg
Males: 11 years and over	18 mg
Females: 11–50 years	18 mg
Females: 51 years and over	10 mg
Pregnant and nursing women	an *extra* 30–60 mg

Effects of Iron Deficiency

A deficiency of iron results in anemia, which is evidenced by pale skin and mucous membranes, weakness, fatigue and shortness of breath due to lack of oxygen. However, the problem is that not all anemia is associated with lack of sufficient iron; therefore, not all anemia will respond to additional iron intake, either in pill form or in the diet. Anemia can be due to lack of vitamin B_6, vitamin B_{12} (pernicious anemia), bleeding from anywhere in the body, protein deficiency, and liver and kidney failure, as well as to certain diseases such as sickle-cell anemia, thalassemia (common in people of Mediterranean origin) and the anemias that can be secondary to problems of the bone marrow and the spleen. Women lose iron through menstruation. Iron deficiency anemia is a major health problem among women of childbearing years. Often their iron requirements cannot be met through the average American diet, and a supplement may be advised. During pregnancy, there is an increased need for the mineral, and the use of 30 to 60 mg of supplemental iron is recommended.

Effects of Excessive Iron

In babies iron and copper are stored in the liver, and the liver makes proteins to store these substances in the blood. If these storage proteins fail to work properly, the baby absorbs excessive amounts of these substances, and it is thought that infantile autism (a mental disorder) might be related to this.

An excess of iron can be serious or even fatal in people with Parkinsonism, sickle-cell disease, hemosiderosis, cirrhosis and thalassemia, among other diseases.

Some schizophrenics also react poorly to excessive iron, as do many with arthritis. Iron deposits are found in the joints of arthritics, and excessive iron may be the cause of bleeding into the joints. At the same time, arthritics have low serum iron, which zinc and manganese supplements may help, since they move iron from the joints to the blood.

Excessive iron can combine with, and prevent proper utilization of, vitamin C, even to the extent of causing scurvy. Children can get an accidental iron overload by swallowing iron supplements, and cooking in iron pots can also increase iron in the diet. Sometimes this is desirable, but the Bantu people of Africa who made a highly acid drink in iron pots ended up developing hemosiderosis (iron overload in the blood). As with other metals, excess iron can gradually be absorbed, and it may take years before the signs of overload become evident. An excess of iron supplements, excessive intake of red wine, excess iron in water

TABLE 8.2
IRON IN SELECTED FOODS

Food	Quantity	Milligrams
Almonds, shelled	1 cup	6.1
Almonds, slivered, not pressed down	1 cup	5.4
Apricots, dried, uncooked	1 cup	7.2
Beans, baby lima, cooked	1 cup	4.7
Beans, pea (navy)	1 cup	5.1
Beef, ground, broiled, lean (10% fat)	3 oz.	3.0
Beef, roast, lean	3 oz.	4.4
Bran flakes, with raisins, sugar, salt, iron, vitamins added	1 cup	16.9
Cashew nuts, roasted in oil	1 cup	5.3
Chili con carne with beans, canned	1 cup	4.3
Chop suey with beef and pork	1 cup	4.8
Clams, raw	3 oz.	5.2
Filberts (hazelnuts), chopped	1 cup	3.9
Heart, beef, lean, braised	3 oz.	5.0
Liver, beef, fried	3 oz.	7.5
Oysters, raw	1 cup	13.2
Peaches, dried, uncooked	1 cup	9.6
Peas, blackeyed, cooked	1 cup	3.5
Prunes, dried, cooked	1 cup	3.8
Pumpkin and squash kernels, dry, hulled	1 cup	15.7
Spinach, cooked	1 cup	4.0
Sunflower seeds, dry, hulled	1 cup	10.3
Walnuts, black, chopped	1 cup	7.5

SOURCE: Adapted from L. Patrick Coyle, *The World Encyclopedia of Food* (New York: Facts On File, 1982), pp. 432–475.

from old pipes and very low-protein diets (vegetarians beware) can also cause iron overload.

The symptoms of iron overload (particularly common in older men) are grayish skin from iron deposits, iron deposits in the organs (liver, heart, pancreas, lungs), dizziness, shortness of breath, weight loss and fatigue.

Meeting Iron Needs

Liver, kidneys, red meats, egg yolks, green leafy vegetables, dried beans, peas, blackstrap molasses, and enriched and whole grains are good sources of iron. Eating foods rich in vitamin C at the same time can increase iron absorption (a double-edged sword in some instances), and use of iron pots can also increase iron intake. Whole wheats contain usable iron, while the form in which iron is added to foods (ferric rather than ferrous iron) can preclude proper absorption.

Iron Supplements

Many iron supplements also contain copper and probably should not be used because excess copper can cause problems. If iron supplements are needed (pregnancy, nursing, periods of rapid growth such as infancy, childhood and adolescence) consult your doctor, since the problems of iron overload may be a consideration, and the "need" for iron may indeed be a "need" for something else in the diet—e.g., an anemia might be due to a number of conditions unrelated to iron intake.

Zinc

Zinc is rapidly becoming a dietary superstar as more and more is discovered about its role in the body. It is known to be vital for DNA and RNA synthesis and is important in the synthesis of over 100 enzymes. It is important in the development of certain eye tissues that enable vision in dim light; it is vital for the development of certain white cells in the immune system; it is necessary for proper gastrointestinal function, for healthy skin, normal growth and functioning of the reproductive system, and normal development of the fetus and the central nervous system; and it is important in blood circulation and clotting.

RDA

Infants: up to 6 months	3 mg
6 months to 1 year	5 mg

Children: 1–10 years	10 mg
Males and females: 11 years and over	15 mg
Pregnant women	an *extra* 5 mg
Nursing women	an *extra* 10 mg

Effects of Zinc Deficiency

Lack of zinc is actually quite common, although borderline deficiency is more common than frank deficiency. Infantile or small sex organs, short stature and anemia are the more obvious symptoms. The development of stretch marks not only in pregnancy but in young people during periods of rapid growth or with exercise, development of painful joints with poor circulation in young people, retarded wound healing, a loss of taste (seen particularly in old people), birth defects, male impotency, excessive copper in the diet, possibly the white spots and white lines in the fingernails and behavioral problems are among those in which a zinc deficiency has been implicated. Persons with liver disease and alcoholics are likely to be more at risk for deficiency, as are those with cancer, intestinal disorders, rheumatoid arthritis and other arthritic diseases, kidney disease, cystic fibrosis and certain inherited skin diseases. People with extensive burns and those receiving steroid medication and anticancer drugs are also likely to be zinc-deficient.

Since zinc is a water-soluble mineral, excessive rainfall can deplete the soil, as can over-planting. This is common in Egypt, Iran and Iraq, where zinc deficiency is very common. Food processing also removes zinc. "Junk food" is virtually lacking in zinc, and this can be very important, particularly for young males. Stress increases the need for zinc, and since zinc is important for the transmission of impulses in the brain, low zinc accompanied by excessive copper may be responsible for such confused states as senility and perhaps some psychotic behavior.

It is sometimes difficult to say whether symptoms are due to zinc deficiency or to something else, but if they respond to supplementation with zinc (under a doctor's supervision, please!), then it is assumed that zinc deficiency was the cause.

Effects of Excessive Zinc

Too much zinc can be as bad as too little, as is the case with most substances. Abdominal pain, anemia, fever and bleeding in the stomach can result. Pregnant women can abort spontaneously or give birth prematurely. Copper deficiency can occur, as well as atherosclerosis (clogging of the blood vessels), nerve damage and muscle weakness.

Meeting Zinc Needs

Meat, liver, eggs and poultry, seafood (particularly oysters) and whole grains are good sources of zinc. Although whole grains are rich in zinc, other substances in grain can prevent absorption. Calcium impairs absorption, but lactose in milk aids absorption, so it about evens out when drinking milk.

Zinc Supplements

Zinc supplementation should only be taken under the care of a physician.

Copper

Copper is essential in the formation of hemoglobin and is a cofactor in many enzymes important for the normal structure and coloration of the hair, the formation of bone and nerve tissue, as well as tendons and arteries and the lungs. Since the amounts of copper required are so small, and copper appears with all the iron salts, plus being a frequent contaminant of food, it is virtually impossible to have a deficiency.

Estimated Safe and Adequate Daily Intake

Infants up to 6 months	0.5–0.7 mg
6 months to 1 year	0.7–1.0 mg
Children 1–3 years	1.0–1.5 mg
4–6 years	1.5–2.0 mg
7–10 years	2.0–2.5 mg
Children and adolescents 11 years and over	2.0–3.0 mg
Adults	2.0–3.0 mg

Effects of Copper Deficiency

In humans only premature infants and those on prolonged intravenous feedings have been found deficient in copper. In animals, symptoms involving virtually every body system can occur— bones, tendons, nerve tissue, major arteries, lungs and hair are defective, and anemia is present.

Effects of Excessive Copper

Copper is considered a heavy-metal intoxicant. Hardening of the arteries, kidney disease, early senility, high blood pressure, psychosis, anemia, heart attacks, violent nausea and vomiting have all been cited as resulting from heavy-metal intoxication, of which copper is one possible cause. Unlined copper pots, copper plumbing (when there is acid water), cigarette smoking and use of oral contraceptives plus stress (which can deplete zinc) can all lead to excessive copper in the body. Food processing that removes zinc, manganese and molybdenum, all of which antagonize copper, further increase the risk of copper poisoning.

Meeting Copper Needs

Oysters, nuts, cocoa powder, liver, kidneys, dried beans and corn-oil margarine are all rich in copper. However, it is hard to find foods without copper. Convenience foods, condiments, sweets and beverages are high, as is wheat germ. So the problem, in many instances, is how to *avoid* copper, not how to *get* it.

Copper Supplements

Copper supplementation is required only for premature babies and hospital patients who are artifically fed. Avoid supplements for other nutrients if they contain copper. Always consult your physician regarding copper supplementation.

Iodine

Iodine is essential for normal reproduction and for production of thyroid hormones, which are important in normal neuromuscular development, rate of bone growth, gastrointestinal motility, development of the cerebral hemispheres (the top, thinking portions of the brain and site of many so-called higher brain functions) and the metabolism of all the cells in the body except the brain cells. Iodine is required for red blood cells and cell respiration.

RDA

Infants: up to 6 months	40 µg
6 months to 1 year	50 µg
Children: 1–3 years	70 µg
4–6 years	90 µg
7–10 years	120 µg
Males and females: 11 years and over	150 µg
Pregnant women	an *extra* 25 µg
Nursing women	an *extra* 50 µg

Effects of Iodine Deficiency

Small deficiencies of iodine cause lethargy, low blood pressure, decreased sexual interest and general slowdown of activity. Goiter (enlargement of the thyroid gland) occurs when the gland attempts to use the small amounts of iodine more efficiently. Many parts of the world lack iodine in the soil, and goiter is very common. Newborns whose mothers were short of iodine develop cretinism, a disorder involving retarded growth, swollen features, protruding abdomen, thick lips and large tongue, accompanied by mental retardation. Persons not eating seafood should use iodized salt, which is sufficient to prevent symptoms in either adults or children.

Effects of Excessive Iodine

Iodine overdosage is not a problem because the body eliminates unused iodine, but some people are sensitive to iodides and develop skin rashes and other symptoms.

Fluorine (Fluoride)*

Fluorine is required for strong bones and teeth. For many Americans fluoridated water is the chief source of this mineral. Although fluoridation has been taking place for many years now, the practice still remains controversial. Despite its success in decreasing tooth decay, opponents of the practice point out that in large doses it can mottle the teeth and may even cause decay. Higher doses can cause brittle bones and very large doses can result in death. (Fluorine was used as a component of nerve gas during World War I.) (For further information, please refer to the discussion of water fluoridation in chapter 10.) Additional sources of fluorine are fish, cheese and meat as well as beverages made with fluoridated water.

Estimated Safe and Adequate Daily Intake

Infants: up to 6 months	0.1–0.5 mg
6 months to 1 year	0.2–1.0 mg
Children: 1–3 years	0.5–1.5 mg
4–6 years	1.0–2.5 mg
7 years and over	1.5–2.5 mg
Adults	1.5–4.0 mg

*Fluoride is the term for the ionized form of the element fluorine, as it occurs in drinking water. Fluorine and fluoride are used interchangeably.

Chromium

Chromium is required for the metabolism of glucose. It is found in meat, cheese, whole grains, dried beans, peanuts and brewer's yeast. Possible abnormal sugar metabolism and adult-onset diabetes may result from a lack of the mineral. Scientists do not know the effects of excessive doses.

Estimated Safe and Adequate Daily Intake	
Infants: up to 6 months	.01–.04 mg
6 months to 1 year	.02–.06 mg
Children: 1–3 years	.02–.08 mg
4–6 years	.03–.12 mg
Males and females: 7 years and over	.05–.20 mg

Selenium

Selenium is required to break down fats and other body chemicals. Seafood, whole-grain cereals, meat, egg yolks, chicken, milk and garlic are good sources of the mineral. Scientists have not yet detected a deficiency of selenium in humans; but animals lacking it suffer from degeneration of the pancreas. Animals given an overdose of the mineral become blind, lame, lose their hair and die; these symptoms have not been seen in humans.

Estimated Safe and Adequate Daily Intake	
Infants: up to 6 months	.01–.04 mg
6 months to 1 year	.02–.06 mg
Children: 1–3 years	.02–.08 mg
4–6 years	.03–.12 mg
Males and females: 7 years and over	.05–.20 mg

Manganese

Manganese plays a number of vital roles in the body, including proper functioning of the nervous system, formation of normal bone structure and maintenance of normal reproduction. It is a part of many important enzymes and also aids in the utilization of fats and in the proper functioning of the liver, pancreas and the adrenal glands. The effects of a manganese deficiency in humans are not known. Excessive doses of the mineral are associated with a masklike facial expression, blurred speech, spastic gait, involuntary laughter and hand tremors.

Estimated Safe and Adequate Daily Intake	
Infants: up to 6 months	0.5–0.7 mg
6 months to 1 year	0.7–1.0 mg

Children: 1–3 years	1.0–1.5 mg
4–6 years	1.5–2.0 mg
7–10 years	2.0–3.0 mg
Males and females: 11 years and over	2.5–5.0 mg

Molybdenum

Molybdenum is part of an enzyme called xanthine oxidase. It is found in legumes, cereal grains, liver, kidneys and some dark green vegetables. No deficiencies have been identified in humans, but animals may have a decreased life span. Loss of copper and a goutlike syndrome have been seen resulting from overdoses.

Estimated Safe and Adequate Daily Intake

Infants: up to 6 months	.03–.06 mg
6 months to 1 year	.04–.08 mg
Children: 1–3 years	.05–.10 mg
4–6 years	.06–.15 mg
7–10 years	.10–.30 mg
Males and females: 11 years and over	.15–.50 mg

Other Trace Minerals

Bromide, cadmium, vanadium, tin, nickel and aluminum as well as silicon have been cited as trace elements found in the body, but to date no recommendations have been made regarding their usefulness or the amounts required. Since they are trace elements, presumably we receive them along with other foods, and if there are any specific disorders associated with either their deficiency or excess, we are not aware of them. In due time, they will make their debut on the dietary scene.

Lead, mercury and cadmium (one of the trace elements mentioned above) are all heavy metals, which can cause severe poisoning and death. Copper, one of the mineral nutrients, has also been implicated when used to excess.

The Bottom Line on Minerals

Perhaps one of the most important considerations about minerals in the diet is the fact that they work together. Both excessive amounts and insufficient amounts tend to disturb the balance of other minerals and vitamins as well as the larger nutrients—the fats, carbohydrates and proteins. In short, the diet must literally be "well balanced" to ensure optimal health.

You should know if the water supply in your particular area is "hard" or "soft" and what minerals are found or are lacking in your area. In times of rapid growth, you should consult your doctor about the need for mineral supplementation—and at all times beware of copper and heavy-metal overload. Iron? Yes, it may be needed—but ask your doctor first. Most mineral supplementation should be taken under medical guidance.

Chapter 9

Salt

Salt is probably the oldest and most widely used condiment and food preservative. The salt mines around Salzburg, Austria have been worked since prehistoric times, and fish preserved in salt was placed in ancient Egyptian tombs. Salt is an ingredient in recipes from every corner of the globe and has been used as a symbol of purity, status and wealth.

Yet lately this commonest of condiments has come into disrepute. Marietta Whittlesey's book, *Killer Salt,* compares "salt addiction" to drug addiction. Others advise eliminating salt from the diet to cure premenstrual tension, kidney stones, depression and other ailments. And reduction or elimination of salt from the diet is medically recommended for patients with high blood pressure.

Are we sickening from an overdose of "lethal crystals," as some writers maintain? Or is salt a necessary ingredient in the human diet? Who should avoid salt entirely? And how—in the age of the fast-food eatery and the quick-mix kitchen—can we reduce our salt intake?

How Salt Works

The chemical name for salt is sodium chloride, a merger between two very common elements, sodium and chlorine. The sodium makes up 40 percent by weight of the total and is the "active ingredient" in salt. It controls the amount of extra water in the body.

Life on Earth began in the salty seas, and even today, all our tissues swim in briny fluid. If you've ever cut your lip or kissed away someone's tears, you know that blood and tears are salty. Some sodium chloride is essential to all of us, and our existence depends on careful maintenance of the proper degree of salinity.

Maintaining the brininess of our internal ocean is the job of our kidneys. If salt intake falls to nothing, they conserve salt. If salt intake zooms, they excrete half the excess in the first day and the rest over the next three days or so. They need a lot of water to take care of a sodium overload, like a bowl of salted peanuts. That is why many bars have those little bowls that indirectly encourage you to drink more. (Unfortunately, the body also needs water to metabolize and excrete alcohol. If you are thirsty, water will slake your thirst better than mixed drinks. And leave the pretzels alone.)

Hypertension

Hypertension isn't nervousness or "that jumpy feeling." In fact, most people with hypertension have no symptoms at all. *Hypertension* is the medical term for high blood pressure.

When a doctor wraps that black rubber cuff around your arm and squeezes it full of air, he or she is measuring your blood pressure with a device called a sphygmomanometer. It measures how hard the blood rushes through your arteries, first when the heart is pumping, and then in the lull between heartbeats. The result is expressed as two numbers signifying the systolic and diastolic blood pressure, respectively. The normal range is 100–140 for systolic and 70–90 for diastolic blood pressure. Authorities differ, however, about the level at which therapy must begin.

If your blood pressure is below this range, but you are otherwise healthy, your doctor will be pleased. Twenty years ago, patients were sometimes given medication to "cure" low blood pressure, but then it was found that low blood pressure is not necessarily a problem. Long-distance runners and other people in top physical condition often had very low blood pressure.

But if your blood pressure is higher than normal for your age, your doctor will probably warn you about the possible consequences of hypertension. When the blood rushes through the arteries too hard, it damages delicate organs: the brain, the heart and the kidney.

The kidney, as explained earlier, is the chief regulator of sodium in the body. Hypertension can damage this mechanism, leading to more sodium retention and further kidney damage. This vicious circle is part of "malignant" hypertension—a leading cause of kidney failure. Often the damaged kidney must be surgically removed to stop the rise in blood pressure.

The heart is even more likely to be affected than the kidney. Common results of high blood pressure are congestive heart failure, heart attack and angina pectoris.

The brain is also vulnerable to the ill effects of high blood pressure. Hypertension frequently precipitates strokes; and headaches, ringing in the ears and dizziness are often symptoms of high blood pressure.

Visual disturbances, due to damage of the blood vessels in the retina (the window of the eye), are another symptom of hypertension.

But people with hypertension may have no symptoms at all, and many Americans have the disease and are unaware of it.

The Salt-Hypertension Connection

Studies of people on high- and low-sodium diets throughout the world seem to indict salt as a precipitating factor in the development of high blood pressure. Where people eat a lot of salt, high blood pressure is common. In Japan, for example, most people eat about three teaspoons of salt per day, mostly in the form of fish, pickled vegetables and soy sauce. In the farm villages of northern Japan, where salt is also used to preserve foods, hypertension can afflict as much as 40 percent of the population. Stroke—often a consequence of high blood pressure—is a leading cause of death in Japan.

Other evidence comes from studies of primitive peoples living simple lives with little or no salt in their diets. These people very rarely have high blood pressure, nor does their blood pressure rise with age, as it does in industrialized countries. (Of course, the tribal peoples of New Guinea, the Amazon basin, Malaysia and Uganda lead very active lives by our standards. This factor might also contribute to the virtual absence of high blood pressure from their societies.)

The classic study linking salt to hypertension took place in the Solomon Islands in the South Pacific. A team of scientists under Dr. Lot B. Page of Harvard, now chief of medicine at Newton-Wellesley Hospital in Massachusetts, studied six tribes whose lives differed significantly by only one factor. Although the lack of roads, telephones and other modern conveniences ensured that all six had plenty of exercise, in three of the tribes, blood pressure increased with age, as it does in industrialized societies. Why? These three ate imported Western foods: salty canned ham and beef jerky. Blood pressure was highest in the tribe that also cooked its fish and vegetables in sea water.

Thus, if you have high blood pressure your doctor may prescribe medicine to lower it. If you are overweight, a diet may be what the doctor orders. But if your blood pressure is even a little higher than normal, he or she will probably suggest reducing the salt in your diet.

Who Has Hypertension?

Estimates of the incidence of hypertension range from 10 million to 60 million people in this country alone. Although the reasons have yet to be determined, black people have twice the susceptibility of others. Hypertension is as common in men as in women, but men seem to be more vulnerable to its ill effects.

Is hypertension inherited? No one really knows. Experiments with animals indicate that a susceptibility to high blood pressure is genetically transmitted, but the most closely related factor is salt intake. Repeated studies have shown that the younger an animal begins to eat salt, the sooner high blood pressure begins. The longer salt is eaten, the higher the blood pressure rises. And the more salt the diet contains, the younger the experimental animal will die.

In addition to salt-intake problems that may be related to racial or hereditary factors, pregnant women and women about to start their menstrual periods often suffer from puffy, bloated hands and ankles. Stimulated by hormone levels, their tissues are retaining extra water—sometimes as much as 5 or 10 pounds of it—all over the body. The problem may be exacerbated by a craving for salt—the proverbial craving of pregnant women for pickles.

The problem is not merely cosmetic, even though it forces some women to acquire two sets of clothes. The excess water can contribute to hypertension (a serious complication in pregnancy) and premenstrual irritability.

If you suffer from either of these complaints, you might try reducing the salt in your diet. (Pregnant women should, of course, modify their diets only under medical supervision.) But the woman who gains weight every month might try reducing her salt comsumption for 10 days before her period begins. It's completely safe, effective therapy, without the side effects of over-the-counter or prescription diuretics often used for this condition.

Is Reducing Salt Intake Safe?

The answer to the question of cutting down on salt is: Probably yes, it's safe. Most Americans eat 2,300 to 6,900 mg of salt per day, about two to three times the minimum daily requirement of 900–2,700 mg. The kidneys are such effective conservers of sodium that even if no salt were ever added to food—as in the diets of some primitive peoples—we could extract enough sodium from meats, fruits and vegetables.

What about those salt tablets people used to take on hot days? They've gone the way of leeches and sulfur-and-molasses tonics. Of course, perspiration is still salty, but the average person would have to sweat at least three quarts—six pounds—before a sodium deficiency developed. So unless you begin a new career digging ditches in the tropics and literally sweating by the bucketful, you don't need salt tablets.

(The dizziness you may feel after exertion on hot, humid days is more likely to be caused by dehydration. You will need to replace the water you have lost. Some self-styled "experts"—athletic coaches, in particular—seem to think that drinking water during exercise is bad for you. At most, they say, you might suck an ice cube for liquid refreshment. These people are wrong. Water restriction during exercise in hot weather has been linked with heatstroke and even death.)

Shaking the Salt Habit

Salt reaches us in three stages: during the processing that takes place before food gets to the supermarket, during cooking and at the table. Let's take them in reverse order.

Salt at the Table

The easiest method of salt reduction consists of not salting before you taste. Salt has no smell, so there is no way a person can tell that a dish needs salt without tasting it. And when you think about it, it's a bit insulting to whomever cooked the food. You wouldn't say to a host or hostess, "I can tell just by looking at this casserole that you left something out." Yet that's the implied meaning of the automatic grab for the saltshaker.

If this doesn't work, remove the saltshaker from the table. Hide it in the kitchen. Around the Mediterranean, many dinners come with a thick slice of lemon. Squeezing this over your meal will give you something to do with your hands—and your taste buds—instead of reaching for the shaker.

Salt in the Kitchen

If you cook for yourself and your family, congratulations! You can control the amount of salt you all eat more easily than anyone else. How? By making your meals from scratch and eliminating the salt from most recipes or reducing it sharply.

This is a big job, especially nowadays when so many people first begin to think about cooking dinner after returning from work at 6 p.m. But unfortunately, almost all convenience foods—frozen, canned, fast takeout—contain much more salt than their homemade equivalents. Luckily, the simplest methods of preparation—without elaborate sauces—generally have the least sodium.

If you already cook from scratch, try halving the salt in those old family recipes. For the first few weeks, the food may taste bland. Not tasteless, bland. Then your taste buds will adjust to the new level of salt, and everything will taste fine again. You can then try a further reduction, if you want to. You can also entirely eliminate salt from dessert recipes without anybody's noticing.

When you buy a new cookbook, compare its recommendations on the use of salt to your own cooking standards. You may need to halve the salt in all of its "old family recipes," too.

There are many ingredients besides salt to enhance the taste of foods. Fresh parsley and other herbs, spices, wine (not "cooking wine"—it contains salt), fresh onion and garlic, and lemon juice will all improve the taste of food without adding significantly to your salt intake.

You will also want to learn the art of making careful and selective choices when you do your grocery shopping. For instance, milk and milk products such as cheese are high in sodium. Your mother told you to drink your milk, but if you want to cut down on sodium, it's time to stop. You can live perfectly well without it if you get your calcium and other nutrients found in milk from different sources. In fact, many black, Oriental and Jewish adults cannot tolerate milk at all. Despite this intolerance, their diet is perfectly adequate.

Other foods that are especially high in sodium are preserved meats—ham, bacon, smoked tongue and all kinds of sausages and luncheon meats like salami, bologna and frankfurters. Shellfish are also high in sodium, as are canned, salted and smoked fish—anchovies, sardines, caviar, smoked herring.

Other very salty foods that you might want to avoid include olives; sauerkraut; condiments like soy sauce, catsup, Worcestershire sauce; pickles and relishes; and party foods—salted popcorn, nuts, potato chips and all the other bright yellow munchies out of cellophane bags. Canned vegetables and soups as well as many fast foods and highly processed foods such as "TV dinners" can also be high in sodium.

Salt at the Processing Plant

About half the salt in the American diet is added by the manufacturers of processed foods—canned and frozen vegetables, soft drinks, processed meats, baked goods, instant dessert mixes of all kinds, breakfast cereals, canned and dehydrated soups and, worst of all, baby foods.

Babies are born with no liking for salt, and their natural food, mother's milk, is very low in sodium. However, many manufacturers salt their baby foods and formulas, and not for the good of the baby. As explained under "Who Has Hypertension?" the earlier a young animal begins to eat salt, the sooner it will develop high blood pressure. But the makers of baby foods want them to be palatable to the mothers, who are reluctant to feed the baby anything that seems "tasteless" because of insufficient salt.

If you want low-sodium food for your baby, you have two choices. One is to puree some of your own food—before you add any salt—in a blender or hand-held baby food grinder. This is probably less expensive than using commercial baby food, although it is sometimes inconvenient to withhold the salt your own palate demands until after the food is cooked. On the other hand, you won't be spending money on innumerable little glass jars.

The other approach is to look for brands of baby food, like Beech Nut, made without salt. In fact, in the last five years, Americans have become more and more aware of the inadvisability of automatically adding salt to *all* foods, not just baby foods. A recent national survey indicated that 40 percent of us are trying to reduce our salt intake. Not suprisingly, manufacturers of convenience foods for adults have followed the lead of baby food makers and are beginning to send low-salt versions of their most popular products to your supermarket.

While the salt-free anchovy pizza has yet to be developed, many all-American favorites are now available in low-salt forms. Salt-free (sweet) butter, always preferred by gourmets, has been joined by salt-free margarine. Canned soups, among the saltiest of foods, are now available in low-sodium versions from Campbell, and no-salt granola and cornflakes can replace more highly seasoned cereals. Salt-free potato chips are just as crisp as salted ones. And saltless or low-sodium peanut butter has spread from the health food store to the supermarket. There is even a low-salt soy sauce, although it is still too salty for people medically restricted to a salt-free diet. You can also look for low-sodium breads in the frozen foods section of your supermarket.

Sometimes these products sit next to their "salty" versions. In other markets, they are in a special section. The most important rule for finding low-sodium products is to read the label. By the start of 1983, under pressure from Arthur Hull Hayes, Commissioner of the Food and Drug Administration, one-third to one-half of FDA-regulated foods will have the sodium content on the label. However, many legislators feel that voluntary measures are insufficient. A bill requiring sodium and potassium labeling of processed and canned foods was introduced in the House of Representatives early in 1982. It would apply to all canned and processed foods regulated by the Food, Drug and Cosmetic Act whose sodium content was more than 35 mg.

If Your Doctor Prescribes a Low-Sodium Diet

The foregoing suggestions are for people who want to reduce their salt consumption to prevent the development of hypertension. What about those whose blood pressure is already too high and whose physicians have recommended a strict low-sodium diet?

If the prescription comes in the form of a complete diet plan, like "Your 1000-Milligram Sodium Diet," a booklet from the American Heart Association, the dieter need only follow it. This may be difficult, but less so than living with the aftereffects of heart attack or with kidney failure.

Unfortunately, not every physician is knowledgeable about which foods contain sodium. All too often, patients are given vague or insufficient—or even contradictory—advice. If in doubt the patient should contact a reliable registered dietitian.

One elderly lady was told by her physician to avoid salty foods. "But what about watermelon pickle? I make it myself. It's my favorite." He agreed to let her have that one condiment. She then proceeded to cut enough thin slices of watermelon pickle to cover everything she ate. This was *not* a low-sodium diet.

Other people convince themselves that sea salt is less harmful than ordinary salt. This is not true. All salt was originally sea salt. Nor are kosher salt, onion salt, garlic salt, seasoned salt, MSG (monosodium glutamate), soy sauce or kelp advisable for people who must reduce their sodium intake.

Foods High in Salt

Foods to avoid include buttermilk (unless you can find unsalted buttermilk), all kinds of commercial foods made from milk, such as frozen desserts, milk drinks and condensed milk. All canned vegetables as well as frozen vegetables processed with salt may also be off limits. Many vegetables may also be forbidden in any form: artichokes, beets and their greens, carrots, celery, Swiss chard, greens like dandelion and mustard greens, spinach and kale, and turnips.

All fresh fruits are fine, in moderation. Starches are a problem, at least in the form commercially available. The only low-salt cereals recommended are "old-fashioned" (slow-cooking) hot farina, grits, oatmeal and wheat cereals, puffed rice, puffed wheat and shredded wheat. Self-rising flour and cornmeal are forbidden, as are salted popcorn, potato chips and pretzels.

Besides the canned, salted or smoked meats and fish and shellfish listed earlier, the person on a low-sodium diet should avoid brains and kidneys and frozen fish. Except for unsalted cottage cheese, all cheeses should be the low-sodium dietetic kind. The same rule applies to peanut butter.

Commercial salad dressings and mayonnaise are off limits, as are bouillon, celery seed, sodium cyclamate, prepared mustard (however, you can easily make your own with dry mustard and water) and horseradish. Almost all commercial condiments—barbecue sauce; catsup; chili sauce; meat extracts, sauces and tenderizers; soy and Worcestershire sauces; and cooking wines—are too salty. They may also contain MSG, another source of sodium.

Non-Salt Sources of Sodium

Salt is not the only danger to the person on a low-sodium diet. Many other food additives—you may have some of them in your kitchen now—contain enough sodium to sabotage a low-sodium diet. The following are among the most common.

Monosodium glutamate is sold under many brand names and in many precooked foods and mixes. It's responsible for the well-known "Chinese restaurant syndrome"—the feeling of aching head and wooziness that many people get after eating in Chinese restaurants. MSG is a flavor enhancer—it doesn't make food taste better, it just makes it taste more, the way a stereo played a little louder sounds a little better. Chinese restaurants used to add it to foods to freshen the dull taste of canned Chinese vegetables. (Non-Chinese restaurants have been known to use this trick, too.)

Besides being full of sodium, MSG can cause brain damage in infant animals, so it is no longer permissible to add it to baby food.

Baking powder and baking soda are used to make breads and cakes rise. You can buy sodium-free versions at health food stores. And please don't add baking soda to cooking vegetables. It is not only unnecessary but harmful: It destroys the vitamins in the vegetables as well as adding sodium. Use something else for indigestion as well.

Brine—a mixture of salt and water—is used in pickling, cleaning and blanching fruits and vegetables, and in flavoring and preserving corned beef and sauerkraut.

Other common additives are disodium phosphate, sodium alginate, sodium benzoate, sodium hydroxide, sodium proprionate and sodium sulfite. As you can see, the word *sodium* on a label (or the chemical symbol *Na*) should act as a "caution" signal.

Water may also jeopardize a low-sodium diet. Tap water may contain from zero to 1,500 milligrams of sodium per quart—and we need 2 or 2^1/$_2$ quarts (including coffee, tea, juices, etc.) per day. Home water-softening systems increase the sodium in the water. If your water is high in sodium, you might want to drink distilled or bottled water. Soft drinks, both regular and low-calorie, may also be high in sodium.

Even medicines contain sodium: antacids, indigestion tablets, antibiotics, cough medicines, laxatives, pain relievers and sedatives. If you are on a restricted diet, check with your doctor before dosing yourself with any nonprescription home cures.

Also check the label before buying a salt substitute. Some of these contain sodium. If you have any doubt, consult your doctor.

Books and Other Aids

Gourmets are not immune to high blood pressure, and several have written low-salt cookbooks, notably Craig Claiborne, food editor of the *New York Times*. He recommends using fresh vegetables and herbs, garnishing foods with mushrooms, onions and tomatoes.

Besides *Craig Claiborne's Gourmet Diet Book,* other low-salt cookbooks include *Gourmet Cooking Without Salt* by Eleanor Brenner; *Cooking Without a Grain of Salt* by Elma W. Bagg; and *How to Live 365 Days a Year the Salt-Free Way* by J. Peter Brunswick, Dorothy Love and Assa Weinberg, M.D.

The American Heart Association publishes a set of useful booklets. Three of these are detailed prescriptions for diets with three different levels of sodium restriction. They are available with a physician's prescription only. A book, *Cooking Without Your Salt Shaker,* contains down-to-earth recipes without salt. These can be obtained from the local office of the American Heart Association.

Many people with hypertension find instruction and support in courses given at nutrition institutes, hospitals or universities. Teachers discuss cooking methods, supermarket label reading, entertaining and how to eat out, both at friends' houses and in restaurants. Some provide lists of restaurants that prepare low-sodium meals on request. Fellow classmates can offer helpful hints and information as well as support. And if the course is prescribed by a physician, Blue Cross will reimburse the patient.

Another aid comes from Mattel Electronics. It's a pocket calculator that "remembers" how much cholesterol, sodium or calories the user has eaten. You can program your daily limit, punch in what you ingest, and it will beep at you to warn of an impending overdose.

Eating Out

Unfortunately, we can't always have complete control over everything we eat. A sodium-restricted diet can complicate the simple pleasures of eating out, either at the homes of friends or in restaurants.

If your doctor has prescribed a sodium-restricted diet, you can simply explain it briefly in response to an invitation. You need not be embarrassed to suggest that the host or hostess set aside a portion of the food before salt is added. If this is impossible, try to eat as little as possible, or be sure you avoid salt throughout the rest of the day. Other alternatives are to volunteer to bring your own salt-free food or to arrive in time for coffee and dessert. After all, you were invited for your company, not to give your seal of approval to the host or hostess's food.

Restaurants are another problem. Chinese restaurants, kosher delicatessens and southern cooking are off limits to those on a low-sodium regimen. Alas, it's not enough to ask them to withhold the MSG, the pickle or the baking powder biscuit. In other types of restaurants, explain your problem and ask lots of questions. Be assertive to find out what is in the food and whether the chef can omit the salt.

For alcoholic beverages, choose a screwdriver or Scotch and water rather than the saltier bloody Mary or Scotch and soda. Hors d'oeuvres are often very highly salted. Avoid soups, and save your appetite for fresh foods, cooked as lightly as possible. Salad with oil and vinegar is ideal. For the main course, ask for broiled meat, fish or chicken, made to order without salt and with the sauce, if any, on the side.

Traveling can also present problems. One pleasant surprise comes on the plane. Almost all airlines will now provide low-sodium meals if they are requested when reservations are made. If you use a salt substitute, it's wise to carry some with you when you travel, along with some salt-free goodies—breads or crackers—in case you have trouble finding suitable food on the road.

Conclusion

Salt has been a very popular and widely used condiment for centuries. Today, we know a great deal about its contribution to health; in some cases, for example, iodized salt has been a valuable addition to the diet and has helped many to avoid the development of goiter. However, salt has been added to so many foodstuffs in the course of processing and preparation that many of us now tend to ingest too much salt, and the result can be high blood pressure, among other ailments. The word *sodium* on any packaged food should be considered a "caution" signal. Low sodium diets may not be advisable for everyone, particularly those without hypertension, but like most foodstuffs, salt should be used in moderation by most. Those with specific medical disorders, such as high blood pressure, who have been advised by their physicians to restrict their salt intake should of course follow their doctors' advice. For the rest of us, good nutritional sense—and moderation—are the keys to using salt wisely.

Chapter 10

Fluids

It has zero calories. It has zero caffeine. It has no artificial sweeteners. Sometimes it even tastes pretty good.

Although it is rarely mentioned as such, water is the most important nutrient of all—vital to health.and vital to life itself. It is possible, for instance, to survive for several months without eating any food, not so much as a radish or celery stick. The body simply draws on fat, protein and minerals it has stored. Stop drinking water, on the other hand, and life would end in just two to three days.

The Body: A Watery Environment

Solid as the human body appears, internally it is made up of about 65 percent water. Astonishing as it seems, the average adult contains about 45 quarts of water, almost half of it located in the cells. Blood, not surprisingly, is 83 percent water. But even solid tissue such as muscle is 75 percent water. Bone is 22 percent.

Water is essential to all the body's vital functions, including circulation, temperature control, digestion, absorption of nutrients and excretion. Via the blood, water carries nutrients from the food we eat, minerals that control the route of the nutrients and oxygen to the body cells. Water also carries away waste materials, the end products of nutrients, to points where they are excreted from the body in the form of urine, feces, sweat and exhaled breath. Among its other important functions, water acts as a cushioner for the tissues and as a lubricator for the joints.

How Much Water Do We Need?

Water contains dissolved salts. The salts regulate the distribution of water within the body. If we drink too little water, dehydration occurs: The salt becomes concentrated, and water is drawn from the cells in an attempt to dilute it. This, in turn, affects the functioning of the kidneys, for regardless of the amount of water taken in, the kidneys must still excrete a minimum of around 10 ounces a day in order to rid the body of poisonous waste materials.

In general, an adult normally loses about 2¹/₂ to 3 quarts of water every day through excretion and perspiration. The rate at which water is eliminated varies, of course, from person to person, depending on body metabolism. But other factors also affect water loss. During such illnesses as fever, vomiting and diarrhea, the body can lose 4 quarts of water a day or more. Water loss is also accelerated during hot weather and through such vigorous types of exercise as jogging, running, dancing, playing tennis, bicycling and even making love.

Staying healthy, therefore, means ensuring a sensible balance between the amount of water and salts consumed each day and the amount of water lost through excretion and perspiration. Under normal circumstances this means putting back some 2¹/₂ quarts of water each day to replace the amount depleted. While it sounds like a lot, most of us do it without even thinking about it.

We don't usually drink 2¹/₂ quarts of fluid each day to begin with. Most of us drink only about 6 to 8 glasses of liquid. Some of it is in the form of plain water, and some is in the form of juices, milk, soft drinks, soup, coffee and tea. The rest of our fluid comes from two other sources. A portion is derived from metabolic processes within the body: Glucose and fats produce water as they are converted to energy. An additional amount comes from foods that have a high water content. Fruits and vegetables, for instance, are usually more than 80 percent water. Even the weight of a solid food such as bread consists of about one-third water.

Because it's not possible to know exactly if fluid needs are being met, the rule of thumb for good health is to drink eight full glasses of liquid a day. And more than that can only benefit—not harm—you. It's a good idea to drink as much as possible of your intake in the form of plain water. Coffee, tea and cola drinks, for instance, contain caffeine, which can make you edgy and tense (see page 164) and has little nutritional value. Caffeine also acts as a diuretic, which means more liquid has to be consumed to counteract the loss of fluid.

Whenever there's a danger of dehydration—during illness or strenuous exercise, or in a hot climate—increase fluid intake considerably and drink more than enough to simply quench thirst.

Remember, unless your doctor has advised you to limit your

intake of fluids, it is always better to drink too much than too little: Any excess fluid will simply be eliminated from the body.

How Pure Is Our Water?

Water is so essential to life that except in times of drought, we rarely give it a thought. Whether we want it for drinking, showering, watering plants, washing dishes or doing laundry, we just turn on a tap and it's there. But today there is growing concern about our water supplies—both their quantity and quality.

About 106 billion gallons of water are used every day in the United States; approximately 75 percent of this amount goes for agricultural purposes. Around half the people in the United States rely on tap water drawn initially from surface water—rainwater that collects on the Earth's surface in rivers, streams and lakes. The other half use water tapped from ground sources, or groundwater—rainwater that seeps into the Earth and accumulates in stretches of sand, gravel and permeable rock known as aquifers. Groundwater may be found a few feet under the Earth's surface or buried deep beneath it.

Just how pure are these sources of water? For the most part, our water supplies are clean and safe to drink. Since 1974 the Environmental Protection Agency (EPA) has been empowered to set national standards for drinking water and monitor state governments to see that these standards are met.

Nevertheless, cases of contaminated water systems have occurred. The reasons are manifold. To begin with, there is no such thing as "pure" water, except in a scientist's laboratory. Rain picks up dust particles and carbon dioxide as it falls to the ground. Then, too, water naturally contains chemicals that may, in excess, create hazards or, when combined with other chemicals, become harmful to health. Additional dangers include bacteria and other disease-carrying organisms in water; the dumping of industrial and chemical wastes that may leak out of their containers and seep into water supplies; and pollutants such as acid rain, pesticides, raw sewage and fertilizers that may be swept into rivers and lakes by rainwater.

In the normal course of events, flowing water can absorb wastes, disperse and dilute them and naturally cleanse itself. In some cases, however, rivers and lakes have become so overloaded with wastes that their natural self-cleaning properties have been exhausted.

Waterborne Diseases

Water pollution is not new. Waterborne diseases such as cholera and typhoid have been known for centuries, though the link between disease and contaminated drinking water was not discovered until 1854, when an English doctor, John Snow, investigated an outbreak of cholera in London. After Louis Pasteur and Robert Koch discovered that many diseases were caused by bacteria and other microorganisms later in the 19th century, municipal authorities began to use filtration methods to purify water. Then chlorine was found to be an effective way to kill bacteria and viruses. Since 1914 both filters and chlorine have been used at U.S. water treatment plants.

While in the United States cholera and typhoid are now virtually diseases of the past, we do have other waterborne diseases to contend with. Two of the most debilitating are amebiasis, or amoebic dysentery, and giardiasis, both of which are caused by parasitic organisms. Symptoms may include acute diarrhea, fatigue and abdominal discomfort.

Once confined mostly to areas of poor sanitation in tropical countries, amebiasis is now found throughout the world. In 1981, 3,731 cases were reported in New York City alone. Amebiasis may be transmitted by the contamination of water supplies with sewage, contamination of food and water with the fecal matter of infected persons or hand contact with a carrier who has not washed his or her hands after using the bathroom. One of the most effective means of prevention is a high standard of personal hygiene. This is particularly vital in the case of people who work in restaurants or other places where food and water are handled.

Giardiasis is spread in similar ways. During 1979, outbreaks caused by contaminated water supplies were reported in California, Oregon, Pennsylvania, Colorado, Utah and Washington. Once an outbreak is identified, residents are advised to boil their water until further notice. During 1980, 11,000 cases of giardiasis were reported to the Center for Disease Control in Atlanta.

Other bacteria, such as salmonella and shigella, have also been identified in U.S. water supplies.

Fluoride—Help or Hazard?

While waterborne microorganisms can be directly linked to illness, some other health aspects of water are not quite so clear-cut.

For example, take the question of fluoride, which is added to some water supplies to help prevent tooth decay.

Fluoride is a trace mineral that combines with calcium, phosphorus and other minerals and is an important element in tooth and bone formation. Fish and seafood are good sources of this mineral. In some areas fluoride also occurs naturally in both surface and groundwater. The amount found varies, but the most usual levels range from a fraction of parts per million (ppm) of water to 3 ppm. Occasionally, the level may be 8 ppm or higher.

During the 1930s, U.S. Public Health Service dentists made studies in areas where water naturally contained a fluoride level of about 1 ppm. They found that children growing up in these areas had around two-thirds fewer cavities than those living in communities where the water did not contain fluoride. Since then small amounts of fluoride, up to about 1 ppm, have been added to water supplies in some parts of the United States. Today around 100 million Americans drink fluoridated water. Some research has shown that as well as reducing tooth decay in the young, fluoridated water may also reduce the incidence of osteoporosis, a progressive thinning of the bones that causes a high fracture rate among elderly people.

Fluoridation remains a controversial issue, however. Some communities have voted against its use, arguing that not enough is known about how fluoride may affect the body when consumed over a long period of time. Concern has also been voiced about whether it might be linked to cancer. A detailed study by the National Cancer Institute concluded that there was no evidence to suggest a relationship between the two.

The only detrimental effect of fluoride use apparent so far is that staining of the teeth may occur in areas where the natural fluoride level is high. In such communities, the fluoride content of the water is usually lowered.

Heart Disease: Hard Versus Soft Water

The part water may play in the incidence of heart disease is another controversial area. However, while there has been some conflicting data, general research in the United States, Canada, Britain and Finland, among other countries, has shown that death rates attributable to strokes and heart attacks are lower in areas where hard water is used.

Hard water contains calcium and magnesium salts. It is these salts that stop soap from lathering easily and make washing dishes, laundry and hair a chore. On the other hand, these same elements may help prevent heart attacks.

Researchers in Finland, for instance, discovered what appeared to be a regional pattern in deaths from heart attacks: In eastern Finland the rate was nearly twice as high as that in the southwest. After some 30,000 soil tests were made, it was discovered that the soil in eastern areas contained only about 100 mg of magnesium per liter. The level increased gradually in a southwesterly direction until in the southwest itself, where the death rate was lowest, the soil contained an average of 300 mg of magnesium per liter. Calcium and potassium levels were also higher in the southwest.

While there does seem to be a relationship between soft water and heart disease, no conclusive evidence has yet been shown. Some scientists believe that soft water may just be connected with a more basic risk factor, or alternatively, that hard water may contain some yet unknown protective factor. Soft water does have a couple of other strikes against it, though. In areas where water is deliberately softened, the sodium content may be raised. This means that heart and kidney patients living in such areas may be getting too much salt from their tap water. Doctors advise switching to a kind of bottled water that has a low sodium content for drinking and cooking.

Soft water can also be corrosive. As it flows through pipes, it tends to dissolve metals. Consequently, it is a good idea to let soft water run for a couple of minutes before using it for drinking or cooking, thereby clearing out water that has been standing in the pipes.

The Cancer Risk

No question arouses more concern than the known and suspected links between contaminated water and cancer. Chemical wastes are the contaminants causing the greatest worry today. The EPA estimates that more than 75 billion pounds of chemical wastes are being generated in the United States each year and that only 10 percent are stored or disposed of in a safe manner. Even chemicals that were considered safely stored years ago are now showing up in some groundwater. The following three examples show how potentially serious the problem of contaminated water may be.

• In 1978 a three-block area in Love Canal, Niagara Falls, was condemned as a disaster area after it was found that chemical wastes buried in a landfill had seeped into the site. Among the chemicals were a number of known cancer-causing agents. Local residents were found to be suffering from a high incidence of cancer, birth defects, and neurological and respiratory problems.

• A 1974 study linked high cancer rates occurring in New Orleans with water supplies taken from the Mississippi River. It was discovered that naturally occurring chemicals in the water were combining with chlorine, used as a purifier, to produce dangerous compounds known as trihalomethanes (THMs). THMs include known and suspected carcinogens.

The study points up how important it is for chlorine levels to be monitored carefully in water treatment plants. Once thought of simply as a safe and effective way to wipe out microorganisms, chlorine is now shown to be potentially dangerous when combined with some other chemicals.

• Over the last few years scientists have detected a potential cancer hazard in the increasing amounts of acid in our surface waters, particularly in heavily industrialized areas of the eastern United States. The acid is produced as sulfur and nitrogen— released in emissions from factory and car exhausts—combines with oxygen, rises into the air and reacts with water vapor. When it rains, the acid may fall into surface water in what is known as acid rain.

What Can We Do?

Thoughts of acid rain and other water pollution problems are not the kind of spurs we need to make us rush for those eight essential glasses of fluid a day. Yet it is important to keep in mind that the EPA sets standards which define the maximum level of pollutants permitted in drinking water and that these standards are well below the level that can cause harmful effects in people.

New ways of treating water are being tested, but meanwhile community action can help ensure vigilance on the part of state and local governments. Among the things we can do are to contact the local water superintendent to find out the sources of local water supply, how it is treated and tested, and whether it meets federal standards. Those of us who have a cistern or septic tank should make sure it is regularly tested and have water samples checked by local authorities.

One simple precautionary measure to help ensure the safety of drinking and cooking water is to *boil it first*. This will kill most microorganisms and disperse organic compounds. Once you have brought the water to a boil, simmer it gently for around 20 minutes, then cover it and store it in the refrigerator.

While some people install home water filtration systems, EPA tests show that many kinds are inadequate and that they allow the growth of bacteria if the carbon filters are not changed frequently.

An alternative measure, though not without its pitfalls, is to drink bottled water.

Bottled Waters

A few years ago bottled waters were the preserve of gourmet shops and fancy delicatessens. Today, partly because of the concern about water pollution and partly because of clever advertising, it is a multi-million dollar industry.

Dozens of kinds of bottled water are available. All of them must meet federal standards, derived from those used for tap water, except for brands labeled "mineral water" (see below). While mineral water is exempt, it is reassuring to know that the Food and Drug Administration does not allow concentrations of any substances to exceed levels that have been classified as toxic.

Not all bottled waters are the same, and labels can be confusing and misleading. Many bottled waters are actually processed tap water. Since the cost of bottled water can sometimes work out to as much as 25¢ or more a glass, an explanation is helpful.

Still Water
This is non-carbonated water such as tap water and bulk water—the kind stored in large containers and used in offices.

Sparkling Water
This is water carbonated by dissolved carbon dioxide gas. Groundwater used for bottling may be naturally effervescent or the bubbles may be added later. A bottled water labeled "naturally sparkling" is drawn from a naturally effervescent source. However, because carbon dioxide escapes, in many cases it is drawn off at the source and reinjected into the water during bottling. Some sparkling water is tap water carbonated with either natural or manufactured carbon dioxide. People with digestive problems or hiatus hernia should be wary of drinking carbonated water.

Mineral Water
In essence, this is water containing dissolved minerals such as

magnesium, potassium, calcium and sodium. (Other than distilled water, all water is technically mineral water.)

Water labeled "natural mineral water" is usually drawn from a spring and may be still or sparkling. It contains only minerals naturally present. When the word "natural" is not used, the water may be processed tap water and have minerals added to it— sometimes in amounts lower than found in water from municipal tap supplies. In cases where the mineral content of the water is naturally high, minerals may be removed to lower the content.

In California, bottled water can be labeled "mineral water" only if it contains a specified amount of minerals.

Spring Water

This is water that rises naturally to the Earth's surface in the form of a spring. Only water labeled "spring water" actually comes from a spring; other terms such as "spring type" or "spring fresh" can be misleading. Spring water is sometimes processed before bottling, sometimes not. The terms "natural spring water" and "natural spring water bottled directly from the source" indicate that the water is unprocessed.

Seltzer Water

This is water, usually tap water, that is filtered for purification, then carbonated. No salts or other minerals are added.

Club Soda

This is also filtered and carbonated water, usually tap water, but minerals and mineral salts are added to it. The sodium content may therefore be high. It is not recommended for people suffering from high blood pressure or heart disease.

Purity of Bottled Waters

In 1980, *Consumer Reports* magazine surveyed more than three dozen different kinds of domestic and bottled waters. Among other things, tests were made for bacterial contamination; mineral content, including sodium; fluoride; heavy metals such as arsenic and iron; selected pesticides; and THMs.

Happily, the results of almost all these tests were satisfactory. No THMs or pesticides could be detected, no dangerous microorganisms were found and levels of most other substances were well within federal standards.

There were three substances, however, that in a few cases did show up in rather high amounts.

Fluoride. Levels were considered high in five of the sparkling mineral waters tested.

Sodium. Levels were considered high in two mineral waters tested.

Arsenic. The federal standard for this metal, which is found in tiny amounts in many foods and waters, is .05 ppm. While bearing in mind that mineral water is exempt from this standard, levels were considered high in four of the mineral waters tested.

Incidentally, *Consumer Reports* also conducted "blind" taste tests of the bottled waters surveyed, and included one other kind of water—New York City water straight from the tap.

Which one got the votes? New York City tap water.

Popular Beverages: Some Special Considerations

What About Alcohol?

Alcohol has been a part of man's diet since early times. The ancient Egyptians made it, drank it and used it in their feasts, ceremonies and religious rites. So did the Greeks and Romans. Through the centuries, people have also argued about the effects of alcohol, the age at which one should be permitted to drink it and, sometimes, whether it should be allowed at all. Today there are still many social, religious and cultural differences among people over the consumption of alcohol.

Does alcohol have any significant nutritional value? The short answer is no. Alcoholic beverages (beer, wine and distilled spirits—gin, whiskey, scotch, rum, vodka, cognac and brandy) vary in the number of calories they contain , but like the calories in sugar, they are all essentially "empty" calories. They do not supply the body with any nutrients.

Wine and beer do contain some vitamins and minerals, it is true, but in such minuscule amounts that their effect is negligible. In addition, alcohol may act as an "anti-nutrient," interfering with the absorption of vitamin B_{12} and using up stores of two other B vitamins: niacin and thiamine.

In reality, alcohol is a toxic drug. While moderate amounts (one or two drinks a day) can sometimes be beneficial, heavy drinking has very harmful effects on the liver, brain, heart and gastrointestinal tract. It can also increase the risk of cancer, lower sexual performance and aggravate attacks of gout, among other things. Women who drink heavily during pregnancy run the risk of causing serious birth defects in their babies.

In addition, we should all be aware of alcohol's significant contribution to auto accidents. More than one-third of adult pedestrian deaths are due to drunk drivers; overall, drunk drivers are involved in nearly half of the almost 50,000 auto fatalities in the United States.

Most people can enjoy an occasional drink without any harmful effect. But, as with any drug, moderation is the key word.

Coffee, Tea and Cola Drinks

Today, Americans consume about 400 cups of coffee per person annually. Tea is not as popular here as coffee; it's more a British institution. Still, in the mid-1970s it was estimated that we were drinking an average of about 150 cups a year.

Along with coffee and tea, we also consume a vast number of soft drinks, an average of around 600 per person each year. Almost three-quarters of the soft drinks consumed are in the form of cola drinks.

Why are we so addicted to these beverages? It's certainly not because they contain useful nutrients. Coffee and tea have little nutritional value and cola drinks may be downright harmful. Along with artificial flavorings and colorings, they contain sugar, sugar and more sugar—sometimes as much as six teaspoons in one regular serving. And along with the sugar come calories. While coffee and tea are low in calories (black has less than 5 calories a cup), cola drinks range from 90 to 120 calories per 8-ounce glass.

Caffeine: a Stimulant

The fact is we are addicted not so much to the beverages themselves but to the caffeine they contain. Caffeine is a stimulant. It acts directly on the nervous system, affecting both the medulla—the part of the brain that regulates heart rate, muscular coordination and breathing—and the cerebral cortex, which controls thought processes. The result is often an edgy, hyperactive feeling.

While caffeine, like alcohol, may be beneficial in moderate amounts, relying heavily on caffeine-containing beverages can be detrimental. For one thing, caffeine relaxes the muscles of the kidneys and increases urinary output. The diuresis (excretion of water) that follows can result in the loss of certain minerals, such as potassium.

Parents should be aware that children are much more vulnerable to the effects of caffeine and that a single 12-ounce serving of cola may provide them with 40 mg of caffeine or more. Cocoa and chocolate also contain caffeine, though in lower amounts than coffee, tea or cola drinks.

Most experts agree that caffeine should be viewed as a drug. In the last few years, a number of studies have been conducted to determine the role of caffeine in the incidence of certain diseases, such as heart disease, cancer, intestinal disorders and birth defects. To date there is no concrete evidence to show that drinking coffee in moderation increases the risk of heart disease. On the other hand, since caffeine is a stimulant, it can certainly produce heart "palpitations" (a faster heartbeat).

There is also no solid evidence to show that caffeine can cause cancer, although the results of a recent survey in Boston suggested that some cases of pancreatic cancer may be related to drinking coffee (these cancers were not linked to drinking tea, suggesting that some other element in the coffee bean besides caffeine may be the culprit). Further studies are needed to corroborate this initial report.

Caffeine has also been implicated in the development of breast cysts. Doctors advise women with mastitis to cut out caffeine completely.

Most people with "nervous" stomachs and/or stomach ulcers readily admit that coffee can irritate the stomach. Both decaffeinated and regular coffees have been implicated.

Caffeine also crosses the placenta, and thus, the developing fetus may easily be affected. Most physicians today advise pregnant women to avoid sources of caffeine.

Finally, caffeine consumption, especially in the form of six to eight cups of coffee a day, can cause headaches and episodes of anxiety. If you experience such symptoms, your best approach would be to begin by reducing your intake of caffeine to see if you can identify it as the cause of the problem. In many cases caffeine is at least a contributing factor.

Those who must avoid caffeine can turn to decaffeinated coffees. Aficionados of coffee frown on the availability of decaffeinated brands and consider them a rather poor imitation of the "real" thing. But those who have switched generally find their taste buds satisfied—and their nerves intact. Herbal tea is another alternative, although some of these blends may be associated with other problems.

Herbal Teas

Because the word *herbal* sounds pleasant and natural, many

people think herbal teas are among the "purest" forms of beverages; on the contrary, many of them contain strong chemicals that can cause such problems as diarrhea, nausea, vomiting and diuresis.

Remember, herbal teas are made from various plants, and plants are also the source of many drugs. As such, a number of elements used in herbal teas, such as senna leaves and aloe leaves, can cause side effects (in this case, diarrhea). Chamomile, another herb used in teas, can cause allergy, especially in individuals allergic to ragweed.

Sorting out the world of herbal teas can turn into a shopper's nightmare. In general, you should stick to brands that you know are safe; if you want to try something new, read the label carefully. If it doesn't provide sufficient information about ingredients contained in the tea, *don't buy it*—you will be better off with traditional brands.

What Ever Happened to Milk?

Years ago, the words "drink your milk" were as familiar as "clean up your room." But today, with the still-growing popularity of soft drinks, coupled with reports of possible side effects of milk (primarily in adults), milk intake is on the decline.

For those who can tolerate it, milk is a valuable source of nutrients. It contains protein, carbohydrates, vital minerals such as calcium and phosphorus, vitamin D and many valuable B vitamins. While milk fat is generally easy to digest, more than half of it is made up of saturated fatty acids, so people counting calories and trying to reduce fat intake may prefer to drink skim milk.

Whole milk and skim milk are probably the most commonly bought types, although buttermilk and evaporated milk are also widely used. Low-fat milk and filled milk are purchased less frequently.

Today it is easy to review the nutritional content of the milk product you buy; in most cases the nutritional components are listed on the carton. *All* grade A milk is pasteurized (to remove menacing microorganisms). Homogenization, on the other hand, results in the dispersion of the fat globules in the milk—which has nothing to do with pasteurization. Frequently, vitamins A and D are added to whole milk, but in these cases the label must state that the milk is fortified.

Virtually all of the fat has been removed from skim milk, while low-fat milk may contain up to 2 percent fat. Evaporated milk may be either skim or whole; "evaporation" merely describes a process by which almost two-thirds of the water is removed from the milk. Filled milk has had some or all of the milk fat removed and another kind of oil or fat substituted. Although the name buttermilk may conjure up visions of lots of calories, in fact, it is considered a low-fat product, unless whole milk products have been added to it. Creams may be purchased as "heavy," which contains 36 percent fat, or "light," which ranges between 18 percent and 30 percent fat.

Milk Intolerance

Breast milk contains all the nutrients an infant needs, though when breast-feeding is not possible, diluted cow's milk is certainly an acceptable alternative. Even as toddlers, however, many of us develop an intolerance for milk (actually, it is an intolerance for the lactose in milk). Ingestion of milk may result in gas, diarrhea, bloating and stomach cramps. Most adult Americans today don't drink milk regularly; we do "outgrow" it and instead derive the nutritional benefits of milk from such dairy products as butter, cheese, and yogurt.

Other disorders are attributed to milk, such as milk allergy and dental problems in children—due to leaving a bottle filled with milk (or fruit juice) in bed with babies, who don't swallow the milk that's in their mouths; instead, pools of milk form, and tooth decay can result.

Finally, since milk, especially whole milk, contains a high amount of cholesterol (about 33 milligrams per cup) and is high in saturated fat and sodium, patients with heart disease are often advised to avoid milk or to stick to skim milk.

Conclusion

Clearly, it is possible to meet our requirements for fluids by drinking a wide variety of beverages. The important point to recognize is that good health can only be maintained by a regular—and adequate—daily fluid intake. Although coffee, tea, cola drinks and even alcoholic beverages may be used to help meet our daily fluid requirements, they should only be drunk in moderation. Drinking plain water is much more beneficial for health.

Chapter 11

Additives

Contrary to what most people think, the practice of adding chemicals to food is centuries old. Salt, sugar, vinegar, smoke and sodium nitrate were the first and were used as preservatives (as well as for taste). With the advent of processed foods, however, came an explosion in adding chemicals to foods. Since it was felt that no one liked the idea of chemicals being put in food, the word *additives* became the euphemism for any "chemicals" being *added* to food. The irony of not wanting to use the word *chemical* is that every living thing is made up of chemicals—including the food we eat (and for that matter, the human body itself).

So why so much concern about chemicals? For one, some chemicals are naturally occurring—essentially inherent in living organisms. Those don't seem to bother people too much. Other types of chemicals are manufactured (produced in a laboratory). These seem to arouse people's greatest concern. What many people don't know is that just because a chemical is naturally occurring doesn't make it good, and just because a chemical is manufactured doesn't make it bad. The deadliest poison known to man—botulism toxin—is naturally occurring. The botulism bacteria can be found in some soil and, unfortunately, in some foods (if not carefully and properly handled). Most antibiotics, on the other hand, are manufactured, but these chemicals (drugs) have saved countless lives.

In other words, we cannot simply judge a chemical (either naturally occurring or laboratory-produced) to be good or bad based on whether it is of natural or manufactured origin. Each chemical must be evaluated carefully, with the decision regarding its use or nonuse being based on the chemical's proven safety and necessity when added to foods.

What Are Additives and Why Are They Used?

An additive is any chemcial that is *added* to food: to prevent food from rotting, spoiling or becoming rancid; to improve its taste, texture, viscosity (consistency) or appearance; or to fortify or refortify its nutrient value. Some additives are almost chemical matches (synthetic reproductions) of naturally occurring substances but are manufactured—not extracted from anything else. Other additives are actually extracted from naturally existing sources. Then, as noted, there are chemicals invented (if you will) and produced in the laboratory by human beings (and these chemicals are not found in any naturally occurring form).

Today, it would be virtually impossible to meet the food needs of the people of the world without processing foods in large quantities. Think about it. How many self-sufficient people do we know who have their own chickens for eggs and poultry; cows for milk, butter, yogurt and ice cream; a large garden for seasonal fresh vegetables; an orchard containing a variety of trees for fresh fruit; and a convenient lake, stream, ocean or pond for fresh fish? How many make their own cheeses, bake fresh breads and pies, or make other bakery goods from scratch? How many make soups? How many can their own fruits and vegetables? (And even then preservatives must be added.)

The point is, the vast majority of people buy foods that have been grown or raised commercially, then processed, packaged and placed on the store shelves. Whether frozen, refrigerated, canned, bottled or boxed—this is the food we most often eat. If we asked the children of today where milk comes from, many would probably tell us "a carton"—not "a cow"! Eggs come from cartons, too, and chicken, beef, veal and fish all come from the "meat department" or the "frozen-food section." Vegetables and fruits aren't really grown—they're found in the "produce section" in neat little rows waiting to be put in clear plastic bags or brown paper sacks (very rare today). Other edibles come from jars, bottles, cans and boxes. Candy and other items are wrapped!

People have come to expect the availability of vast supplies of an endless variety of foods (no matter what time of year it is)— foods that will be uniform in quality, convenient and safe for consumption.

Without food processing and the use of *some* additives, not all of those things would be possible. Therefore, unless we totally change our expectations and are willing to provide for our own nutritional needs by growing and raising our own food (which is unrealistic at this point), we have to expect that foods will be processed and additives will be used. It is only right, however, that the consumer also expect that the additives put into foods will be safe and necessary. (We will discuss safety and necessity later in this chapter.)

The Kinds of Food Additives

There are essentially thousands of different food additives. Their purposes are many and varied. Some of these additives are very useful, while others (many feel) may be questionable. A review of some of the types and purposes of additives will give us a better understanding of what they are and what they do.

Preservatives

As previously noted, food preservatives were used centuries ago. Their purpose then and their purpose now (although many are more sophisticated and effective today) is to prevent food from spoiling or becoming inedible. If food can be "preserved," then it can also be made available throughout the year.

One kind of preservative retards (or stops) the growth of bacteria, yeast and molds (microorganisms) that can poison or destroy food. These additives are called antimicrobial agents. There are some common ones you may be quite familiar with, such as salt, sugar, vinegar, sodium nitrate, ascorbic acid, sorbic acid, calcium and benzoic acid.

Another type of preservative prevents oils and fats from becoming rancid. These additives, which also prevent some fruits and vegetables from turning brown (or discolored) after they are cut, are called antioxidants. The most familiar ones are BHT (butylated hydroxytoluene), BHA (butylated hydroxyanisole), propyl gallate, ascorbic acid (vitamin C) and citric acid.

Emulsifiers, Thickeners and Stabilizers

Have you ever wondered why the water and oil in salad dressings mix so well instead of separating? Why mixtures such as mayonnaise or peanut butter don't separate, are consistently creamy and are thick? Why the chocolate in chocolate milk stays so well mixed with the milk instead of falling to the bottom of the container? Why some canned soups, gravies and so many other edibles are so thick (including boxed foods once milk or water are added)? Why some potato chips, tortilla chips and other chips and crackers are so crisp and not dried out? Or why the texture of instant mashed potatoes is "like" real mashed potatoes?

The answer to all of these questions is often—additives! Emulsifiers are additives that allow the mixing of liquids that would normally separate. Some of the most commonly used emulsifiers are lecithin; mono- and diglycerides; polysorbate 20, 40, 60, 65 and 80; arabinagalactose; propylene monostearate; sorbitan monostearate; and sodium silicate. Stabilizers and thickeners are often one and the same (that is, a single additive that serves both functions) and not only prevent mixtures from separating but add viscosity and texture. Some commonly used stabilizers/thickeners are carob bean gum, guar gum, gum acacia, propylene glycol, sodium methyl cellulose and sodium alginate.

Flavorings and Flavor-Enhancers

Essentially, flavorings or flavor-enhancers are put into food to add or enliven taste. Many natural flavorings are used, as are synthetic reproductions of naturally occurring flavorings and purely chemical inventions. Some flavorings and flavor-enhancers are as common as cinnamon, turmeric, vanillin, paprika and MSG (monosodium glutamate); and others are as unfamiliar as disodium guanylate, disodium inosinate, yeast-malt sprout extract and hydrolyzed vegetable protein (HVP).

Colors

Colors can be either naturally occurring chemicals or synthetic dyes. Color is added to foods to make them more appealing. Some naturally occurring colors include beet powder (dehydrated), beta-carotene, carminic acid, carrot oil, grape skin extract, paprika, riboflavin, saffron, turmeric, titanium and vegetable juice. Presently the synthetic colors approved for use are : Blue No. 1, Blue No. 2, Yellow No. 6, Red No. 3, Red No. 40 and Green No. 3.* Two other colors are approved with very specific restrictions (Orange B and citrus Red No. 2).

The reason so few colors have been certified "harmless" is the Delaney Clause of the Food and Cosmetic Act, which basically says that any additive is absolutely banned if it has produced cancer in laboratory animals. Any new evidence of cancer in animals (or humans) being caused by existing approved colors (or other additives) would result in those colors (or additives) being dropped from the approved list. Most opponents of the use of colorings note that they are used only for cosmetic purposes.

---

*Blue No. 2 is currently under investigation and there have been demands that it be banned. At press time the FDA had not ruled on the substance.

Sequestrants and Acidulants

Basically, sequestrants remove or trap trace metals that can cause food to go rancid or discolor. Common sequestrants are citric acid, sodium metaphosphate and EDTA (ethylenediaminetetraacetic acid). Acidulants have many purposes—as flavorings, preservatives and antioxidants—and are also used to maintain a desired acidity or alkalinity in foods. The most commonly used acidulants are citric acid, acetic acid (vinegar), lactic acid, sodium bicarbonate (baking soda), phosphoric acid and sodium citrate.

Nutrients

Nutrients are added to food for two reasons: (1) to replace the naturally occurring nutrients that were reduced or destroyed during processing and (2) to improve the nutrient value of the food. Some of the nutrients added to food include vitamins, amino acids, potassium iodide, folicin, baker's yeast protein, kelp, aluminum nicotinate and iron choline citrate complex.

Nutritive and Nonnutritive Sweeteners

Nutritive sweeteners are added to food to enhance its taste and/or to increase its caloric content. Some include glucose, dextrose, fructose, sucrose, maltose, honey and maple syrup. Nonnutritive sweeteners are used for taste enhancement and to replace sugar, while adding few, if any, calories. Sodium saccharin is most often used today, but a warning is placed on food and beverage items that reads: "Use of this product may be hazardous to your health. This product contains saccharin which has been determined to cause cancer in laboratory animals." Cyclamate, another artificial sweetener, was banned after studies in rats found that it could cause cancer. Still another nonnutritive sweetener, aspartame, is presently approved for use.

Humectants and Leavening Agents

Humectants are additives that help keep food moist and maintain the desired texture. Commonly used humectants are sorbital, mannitol, glycerine and propylene glycol. Leavening agents are commonly used in baking and are well recognized by most people. Some include sodium bicarbonate (baking soda), baking powder, yeast, sodium aluminum phosphate, sodium aluminum sulphate and calcium phosphate.

Dough Conditioners and Anti-Caking Agents

Dough conditioners are additives that reduce firmness in dough to make it more palatable. Examples include calcium sulfate, ammonium monocalcium phosphate, potassium bromate and benzoyl peroxide. Anti-caking agents are additives that keep powdered mixes (such as seasoning salts) from clumping into solid masses when the climate is damp or there is moisture in the air. Examples include mannitol, calcium silicate, magnesium carbonate and calcium stearate.

Miscellaneous Additives

There are many other kinds of additives used in foods besides the most common ones mentioned above. Some make foods firmer, while others make foods softer. Some make certain foods or drinks foam up, and others make foods or drinks foam down. There are additives for making liquids clearer and additives for making liquids darker. There are even additives to "remove" naturally occurring or other chemicals (the best example being the removal of caffeine from coffee, tea or sodas).

The Risk-Benefit Ratio of Additive Use

As noted earlier, not all additives (whether naturally occurring, extracted or invented) are bad, nor are all good. In the field of health care today, for example, there is a rule of thumb known as the risk-benefit ratio. That is, every medical test to be given, every treatment to be performed and every medication to be prescribed should be evaluated and judged based on its risk-benefit ratio. If the potential benefits outweigh the potential risks, then the test, treatment or medication should more than likely be approved. However, if the potential risks outweigh the potential benefits, then obviously the test, treatment or medication should not be approved.

This same basic principle is in fact applied to most things in society and is a reasonable approach to determining relative safety. But there is one basic premise involved here—relative safety—that few people really understand. When safety is determined in most instances, the judgment of "safe" actually means "relatively safe." But "safe" to most people means no harm can be caused—ever. This is misleading. Nothing is absolutely safe and harmless—100 percent of the time. Driving a car has risks associated with it. Playing a sport has risks associated with it. Even walking across a street or taking a shower have risks associated with them. The point is, all are considered safe, or doing any of those things would be banned out of respect for everyone's safety and well-being. Or, to put it more precisely, all are considered *relatively safe*—that is, the benefits most often outweigh the potential risks.

With additives it must be remembered that any chemical (even water) if used in excess or without respect can result in problems. Therefore, things are judged safe or unsafe based on proper use, not on overuse or abuse. The FDA (Food and Drug Administration) uses three guidelines to determine the relative safety of food additives: (1) If taken over long or extended periods of time—in increasing dosages—does the chemical cause harm (or become hazardous)? (2) Does mixing the chemical with other chemicals cause harm, or could mixing potentially result in harm? (3) Are there appropriate safety factors related to its use?

Although food additives are better tested today than ever before, there are still many controversies surrounding their safety. First of all, there has been some concern over what is called the *GRAS list* or *GRAS substances*. GRAS stands for "*G*enerally *R*ecognized *A*s *S*afe." A little history is necessary in order to understand the significance of this list of substances.

Before 1958 additives could be put into food as long as they were not considered poisonous or unsafe. Although poisonous or unsafe additives (whether naturally occurring or not) were essentially prohibited, the burden of proof that an additive was *not safe* was on the government *after* the additive came into use. The Food Additives Amendment passed in 1958 changed this. After 1958 the burden of proof that an additive was safe was transferred to those who wanted to use the additive in processing. Furthermore, the additive would have to be approved/certified *before* it could be used.

However, this did not apply to chemicals or substances used before 1958. Thus, the GRAS list came into being. Basically, the list was to include "any substance of natural biological origin that has been widely consumed in the United States prior to 1958, without known detrimental effect, for which no known health hazard is known." Therefore, 670 substances were placed on the GRAS list based on any available data (up to that date) or determined by their prior use in foods. In other words, items on the GRAS list would not have to undergo formal testing. However, items could be removed from the list if studies or other new data proved them to be unsafe.

The problem with the food additives issue, some claim, is that people have become unrealistically skeptical or mistrusting. Others argue that there are good reasons for skepticism. For one, in 1980 a group of scientists (independent of the FDA) finished a review of 415 of the substances on the GRAS list and reported their findings to the FDA. These scientists said that 305 of the GRAS list substances were safe; 68 required more information (but were deemed all right); 19 required additional studies because uncertainties existed; 5 required restrictions as currently utilized; and 18 had insufficient or inadequate data to judge. Independent testing and reporting to the FDA is continuing on GRAS substances as well as on those substances approved after 1958.

The Controversies—What Are They?

Besides criticisms of the GRAS list, there have been other controversies surrounding food additives. Here is a concise overview:

- The testing procedures and validity of tests by manufacturers—the results of which are submitted to the FDA for the evaluation and approval of additives—have been questioned.
- There are those who feel that not enough is known about the interaction of additives and other chemicals or substances in food. Something that might be perfectly safe alone may not be when mixed with other substances.
- There are those who feel that certain additives should have been banned outright instead of restricting their use, placing warnings on labels or doing nothing whatsoever.
- There is some suggestion that food additives (particularly food colors) may cause behavioral changes, especially in children.
- Others note that it is difficult to determine whether some so-called food allergies are not in fact allergies or reactions to certain additives instead.

At this point, you are probably asking for a simple solution to the food additive issue. Unfortunately there is no simple answer—no pat "here are all the facts" explanation. This, in part, is why so many controversies surround the use of food additives—there are still many questions to be answered and often no clear-cut "absolutes"—either pro or con. What seems to cause concern is the gray area when it comes to the use or nonuse of products that contain certain additives.

You may be saying, "What about all the controversy I hear about the use of nitrites in hot dogs and bacon? I've heard a lot of talk about the danger of nonnutritive sweeteners. Is there any truth in this? Is it true that flavorings could be dangerous? What about food colorings—do they have any value besides cosmetic? I've heard that DES is still fed to cattle—is that true?" The questions go on and on.

The fact is, no chapter such as this could possibly begin to address all the details of the numerous food additive controversies that have arisen over the past several decades. It is possible, however, to briefly discuss some of the key controversies. Following is a general overview of some of the information available so far about certain additives that have received particular attention by the news media and the general public. (It is very important to remember that research about additives is ongoing, and we must be attentive in order to stay up to date on the status of those being tested.)

BHT and BHA

The abbreviations *BHT* and *BHA* are more often listed on food items than their full names. BHT (butylated hydroxytoluene) and BHA (butylated hydroxyanisole) are preservatives that prevent oils and fats from becoming rancid and are also used to prevent some fruits and vegetables from discoloring or turning brown after being sliced. Many vegetable oils and processed foods with fat or oil in them have BHT and BHA added. Because some companies do not use BHT and BHA and still make quality products, many feel the use of these additives is not warranted. Opponents to their use say BHT and BHA are of little benefit to the consumer and should not be used (most particularly because the two have not been tested specifically to see if they are possible carcinogens).

One general study implicated BHT as a possible cause of birth defects in rats, yet other studies six years later noted that BHT was safe and did not cause birth defects. Some short-term studies (done with rats and dogs) have shown that very high dosages of BHT resulted in enlargement of the liver and the development of high liver enzyme levels (indicating liver damage). The conflict between the studies has led many to feel that, considering the common use of BHT and BHA, they have been inadequately tested. Those who believe BHT and BHA should be avoided can do so by using oils, shortenings, potato chips, candy and other products that do not have these additives in them. (If BHT and BHA have been added, it must be so stated on the product label.)

MSG (Monosodium Glutamate)

A sodium salt of glutamic acid (an amino acid), MSG has an amazing ability to enhance or intensify the flavor of foods containing protein. Initially, controversy arose in 1968 when a doctor discovered what he called "Chinese restaurant syndrome" or "CRS." He reported that approximately 30 minutes after starting a meal at a Chinese restaurant he experienced very strange symptoms—an odd burning sensation in the back of his neck and forearms, as well as headaches and tightness in his chest. The problem was traced back to a soup containing MSG. Later research substantiated his findings.

Chinese restaurant syndrome does not appear to cause any permanent damage. However, one study of infant mice (who received large amounts of MSG) showed nerve cell destruction in the hypothalamus (the area of the brain that controls many important body functions, including regulation of body temperature and appetite control). Other mice and rat studies have shown similar results, with additional evidence of injury to the retina (the tissue at the back of the eye that receives visual images). But still other studies on baby animals (rabbits and chickens) indicated no damage to the brain or other problems.

Until 1969, baby food manufacturers used MSG in their food. After 1969, the manufacturers voluntarily produced foods without MSG because of public demand. However, baby foods containing MSG were still found in supermarkets well over a year later (since existing food was not recalled). The use of MSG in baby foods has not yet been banned, but these additives continue to be avoided in manufacturing.

There is some justifiable concern about use of MSG by expectant mothers. Apparently, the human placenta concentrates MSG, so the fetus might receive a proportionately higher "dose" of the substance than the amount the mother consumed. Although it is believed that the usual expectant mother would not normally consume enough MSG to cause problems for the fetus, many feel it is best for all pregnant women to either avoid its use or be quite prudent in the amount consumed—at least until more extensive studies can be performed and results reported. One note: a 1980 FDA review panel concluded that MSG (as presently used) is not a hazard for adults. They did, nonetheless, recommend that care be taken in the amount added to foods.

Sodium Nitrite and Sodium Nitrate

These additives are used to preserve bacon, frankfurters, ham, smoked fish, processed or cured meats and luncheon meats. They also give these products the characteristic pinkish-red color considered so attractive and appealing. What isn't so appealing is that when nitrites and amines (from proteins) mix—they can form nitrosamines. The problem? Nitrosamines have caused several types of cancers in almost all studies on animals (no matter what species of animal was tested). Bacon treated with nitrite, for example, can form nitrosamines when fried at 370 F or higher.

However, the case against the additive is not conclusive. Only about 20 percent of our daily nitrite exposure is the result of food additives; the other 80 percent of our daily exposure is naturally occurring. If you took one average serving of cured meats and compared that to the nitrite naturally produced in human saliva, for example, you would be amazed to find that human saliva produces almost four times the nitrite you'd get from eating the single serving of cured meat. Nitrates are also naturally found in some vegetables. Digestive juices are able to change a part of the nitrates into nitrites. These nitrites can then potentially mix with other foods to form nitrosamines. Nitrosamines were also found in some beers and scotch tested (probably the result of barley malting). As a result, by January 1980 an alternative processing method was instituted. There may still be "trace amounts" of nitrosamines in these beverages.

Because there is no evidence that nitrosamines in foods have caused any cancer in humans, the FDA has not banned sodium nitrite or sodium nitrate. However, the United States Department of Agriculture did mandate that the amounts of nitrites and nitrates be reduced in some products and eliminated from others.

Meats and fish treated with nitrites-nitrates have all the ingredients to form nitrosamines—the chemical treatment provides the nitrites and the protein in the meats and/or fish provides the amines. Opponents of the additives claim their use in protein-containing products to be the greatest potential hazard and point out that any reduction in exposure to nitrites would be healthier. By removing nitrites and nitrates from foods, we would therefore experience a 20 percent reduction in exposure—to many a significant difference.

Proponents of nitrates-nitrites say there is presently no scientific evidence that these substances cause cancer in humans. They also point out the usefulness of these additives in retarding the growth of botulism and other microorganisms, as well as their flavoring and coloring capabilities.

For those who agree that nitrates and nitrites should be avoided, read the packaging label to determine if these were used in the product. Note specifically the information on bacon, cured or processed meats, ham, sausage, knockwurst, frankfurters, luncheon meats and smoked fish. Those products prepared without nitrites-nitrates are usually labelled "uncured."

DES (Diethylstilbestrol)

DES is a synthetic hormone that was used to stimulate growth in cattle (in particular). This hormone works like estrogen (the female hormone) and is known for its ability to "plump up" (add lean meat more rapidly to) cattle, chickens and other livestock. By using DES, the amount of grain necessary to feed the animals (in order to reach the desired size) was reduced. This then reduced the cost to the consumer.

The problem is that DES is a carcinogen when consumed. For example, when DES was given in large doses to expectant mothers, it was thought to be a safe drug useful in preventing miscarriage. However, many of the daughters of women who took DES during pregnancy have experienced vaginal and/or cervical cancers of an unusual type, while others have experienced abnormal changes in the cervix. The FDA has banned the use of DES because it is a carcinogen, although the manufacturers of the synthetic hormone fought this action. Its use must be avoided, and care should be taken to ensure that DES is never again used.

Certainly there are many other additive controversies than those few discussed. However, these give some idea of the type of controversies that exist and the complexities involved. The more we understand food additives, the better equipped we are to make our own informed judgments regarding the risk-benefit ratio of various additives as they come into question.

Some Additives To Avoid

Table 11.1 provides a list of those additives that should be avoided as well as those that individuals may choose to avoid (based on their own personal risk-benefit analysis) until more information is known; there is also a small section included on the list about "safe additives."

TABLE 11.1

COMMON FOOD ADDITIVES: HOW SAFE ARE THEY?

Avoid

Artificial Colorings: Most are synthetic chemicals not found in nature. Some are safer than others, but names of colorings are not listed on label. Used mostly in foods of low nutritional value, usually indicating that fruit or natural ingredient omitted.

Additive	Use	Comment
Blue No. 1	In beverages, candy, baked goods.	Very poorly tested.
Blue No. 2	Pet food, beverages, candy.	Very poorly tested
Citrus Red No. 2	Skin of some Florida oranges.	May cause cancer. Does not seep through into pulp.
Green No. 3	Candy, beverages.	Needs better testing.
Orange B	Hot dogs.	Causes cancer in animals.
Red No. 3	Cherries in fruit cocktail, candy, baked goods.	May cause cancer.
Red No. 40	Soda, candy, gelatin, desserts, pastry, pet food, sausage.	Causes cancer in mice. Widely used.
Yellow No. 5	Gelatin dessert, candy, pet food, baked goods.	Poorly tested; might cause cancer. Some people allergic to it. Widely used.
Brominated Vegetable Oil (BVO)	Emulsifier, clouding agent. Citrus-flavored soft drinks.	Residue found in body fat; safer substitutes available.

Butylated Hydroxytoluene (BHT)	Antioxidant. Cereals, chewing gum, potato chips, oils, etc.	May cause cancer; stored in body fat; can cause allergic reaction. Safer alternatives.
Caffeine	Stimulant. Naturally in coffee, tea, cocoa; added to soft drinks.	Causes sleeplessness; may cause miscarriages or birth defects.
Quinine	Flavoring. Tonic water, quinine water, bitter lemon.	Poorly tested; some possibility that may cause birth defects.
Saccharin	Noncaloric sweetener. "Diet" products.	Causes cancer in animals.
Sodium Nitrite, Sodium Nitrate	Preservative, coloring, flavoring. Bacon, ham, frankfurters, luncheon meats, smoked fish, corned beef.	Prevents growth of botulism bacteria but can lead to formation of small amounts of cancer-causing nitrosamines, particularly in fried bacon.

Caution

Artificial Coloring: Yellow No. 6	Beverages, sausage, baked goods, candy, gelatin.	Appears safe, but can cause allergic reactions.
Artificial Flavoring	Soda, candy, breakfast cereals, gelatin, deserts.	Hundreds of chemicals used to mimic natural flavors, almost exclusively in "junk" foods; indicates "real thing," is left out. May cause hyperactivity in some children.
Butylated Hydroxyanisole (BHA)	Antioxidant. Cereals, chewing gum, potato chips, oils.	Appears safer than BHT but needs better testing. Safer substitutes available.
Heptyl Paraben	Preservative. Beer.	Probably safe, has not been tested in presence of alcohol.

Monosodium Glutamate (MSG)	Flavor enhancer. Soup, seafood, poultry, cheese, sauces, stews, etc.	Damages brain cells in infant mice, causes "Chinese restaurant syndrome" (headache and burning or tightness in head, neck, arms) in some sensitive adults.
Phosphoric Acid; Phosphates	Acidifier, chelating agent, buffer, emulsifier, nutrient, discoloration inhibitor. Baked goods, cheese, powdered foods, cured meat, soda, breakfast cereals, dried potatoes.	Useful chemicals that are not toxic, but their widespread use creates dietary imbalance that may be causing osteoporosis.
Propyl Gallate	Antioxidant. Oil, meat products, potato stocks, chicken soup base, chewing gum.	Not adequately tested, use is frequently unnecessary.
Sulfur Dioxide; Sodium Bisulfite	Preservative, bleach. Sliced fruit, wine, grape juice, dried potatoes, dried fruit.	Can destroy vitamin B-1, but otherwise safe.

Safe

The following common food additives are rated as safe by the Center for Science in the Public Interest. Space restrictions prohibit a detailed description of each additive. The additives are: Alginate, Propylene & Glycol Alginate, Alpha Tocopherol, Ascorbic Acid, Erythorbic Acid, Beta Carotene, Calcium (Sodium) Propionate, Calcium (or Sodium) Stearoyl Lactylate, Carrageenan, Casein, Sodium Caseinate, Citric Acid, Sodium Citrate, EDTA, Ferrous Gluconate, Fumaric Acid, Gelatin, Glycerin (Glycerol), gums (Locust Bean, Guar, Furcelleran, Arabic, Karaya, Tragacanth, Ghatti), Hydrolyzed Vegetable Protein (HVP), Lactic Acid, Lactose, Lecithin, Mannitol, Mono- and Diglycerides, Polysorbate 60, 65 and 80, Sodium Benzoate,

Sodium Carboxymethyl-cellulose (CMC), Sorbic Acid, Potassium Sorbate, Sorbitan Monostearate, Sorbitol, Starch and Modified Starch, Vanillan, Ethyl Vanilian.

Special Considerations

	Special Considerations
Salt (Sodium Chloride)	Flavoring. Most processed foods: soup, potato chips, crackers, cured meat, etc. Large amounts of sodium may cause high blood pressure in susceptible persons and increase risk of heart attack and stroke.
Sugars: Corn Syrup, Dextrose, Glucose, Invert Sugar, Sugar	Sweeteners. Candy, soft drinks, cookies, syrups, toppings, sweetened cereals and many other foods. Mostly in foods with low, if any, nutritional value. Excess sugars may promote tooth decay and precipitate diabetes in susceptible persons; condensed sources of calories.

SOURCE: Reprinted from Chemical Cuisine poster, which is available from the Center for Science in the Public Interest, 1755 S Street, N.W., Washington, D.C., 20009, for $3 ($6 laminated), copyright © 1982.

Is "Natural" a Hoax?

Some people contend that natural foods contain no additives. But remember, everything is essentially a chemical—even naturally occurring substances are chemicals. The food may not have *laboratory-produced* additives, but it can have other "natural" chemicals. This is not to say that "natural" is a hoax. It's simply a matter of knowing exactly what we are buying. The product may or may not have natural additives in it, and we should be aware of this and read the labels. Also, often very safe and helpful nutrient additives have been withheld from certain foods, just so they could be called "natural." So we should be aware of what nutrients are or are not in the product, too. Just because it is "natural" does not mean it will meet nutritional requirements for particular vitamins, minerals or amino acids. It is always prudent to check the labels of all food purchased.

The Bottom Line on Food Additives

What it all comes down to regarding the often-heard criticism of food additives seems to be an overriding feeling that more extensive, lengthy studies should be performed and that *no additive* should be used that is not absolutely necessary and proved safe. Most people agree that food additives are required to maintain an adequate, proper and high-quality food supply. Their argument is with those additives that are potentially hazardous or unnecessary. Food colors, for example, merely enliven the appearance of food. Many have already been proved unsafe and banned. Others are being studied. Critics question the need for any of them. Proponents say they make food more appealing and appetizing and are therefore necessary. It is cases like this that have caused the public to become increasingly concerned.

The "truth in packaging" laws of 1967 and 1973 established nutrient labeling regulations that work in the consumers' favor. The important thing to remember when shopping is to *read the labels*. Buy foods that have the fewest number of additives and don't buy those with additives whose safety is still in question.

Chapter 12

Putting It All Together

Up to this point we have detailed the various components of good nutrition but have discussed them as separate entities. Carbohydrates, proteins, fats, vitamins, minerals, fiber and water, however, do not work alone. Together they ensure that the body's energy needs and the nutrient requirements of all organs and tissues are met. In a sense, when it comes to nutrition and good health, the *whole* does equal the *sum of its parts!* For the information presented earlier to be useful to you, we must now "put it all together" to reach a formula for excellent nutritional habits.

The Four Food Groups

Nutrition and the body have confused people for a very long time. In an effort to simplify nutritional requirements, the U.S. Department of Agriculture (USDA) developed the concept of the four basic food groups. Although this system was developed many years ago, a lot of people still do not quite understand how and why it works. Essentially, foods were divided into groups based on their nutrient content. If a specific number of servings from each of the four groups were eaten every day, basic nutritional requirements would be met. Serving sizes would be based on energy needs (less active people require smaller serving sizes, and those more active require larger serving sizes). Clearly, structuring your nutritional plan by using the four basic food groups system is reasonable and easy.

However, many people still find this system complex. Part of the problem is that nutritional requirements change at certain times in our lives—for example, as we age, when a woman is pregnant, or even when a chronic illness occurs. These "special requirements" are really not difficult to understand once you have a good grasp of basic nutritional principles.

The four basic food groups concept is still the best and easiest nutritional plan to utilize on a day-to-day basis. Here's what you need to remember. The four basic food groups are:

- Dairy products
- Meats and other proteins
- Fruits and vegetables
- Grains and cereals

(See Table 12.1 for a more detailed list of the foods found in each group.)

By having a certain number of servings from these four basic food groups each day, you can reach a balance of proteins, carbohydrates and fats as well as essential vitamins and minerals. It's really a matter of putting together the correct combinations in the quantity of each needed. The number of servings from each group breaks down like this:

The four basic food groups and the daily recommended servings are excellent *baselines* for meeting nutritional requirements. Serving sizes are then based on overall calorie needs (energy requirements).

In order to determine the number of calories needed daily, you should first determine your ideal weight, based on your height, frame size and sex. (See Table 12.2.) Research has shown that an adult male needs approximately 1,650 calories per day and an adult female 1,350 calories per day to meet the body's "average basal energy requirement." The basal energy requirement represents the number of calories (units of energy) needed per day for normal body metabolism at rest. The basal energy requirement usually represents about two-thirds of a moderately active adult's total daily caloric needs. The other one-third of daily calories should represent those needed to meet energy requirements due to daily activity level. Remember, these recommended caloric intake levels are only averages for the adult male and female and will vary depending on each person's frame size (bone structure), body build (muscular or not), sex, age and metabolic function. As we age, our basal energy requirement decreases, as does our daily activity level (in most cases).

Once you know what your ideal weight is, then you can determine what your total daily caloric intake should be to maintain you at your ideal weight or to gain or lose pounds in order to reach your ideal weight. It takes 3,500 unused calories (units of energy) to produce one pound of body fat. To lose one

TABLE 12.1
FOUR BASIC FOOD GROUPS DAILY INTAKE GUIDE

Milk Group (8-ounce cups)
  2 to 3 cups for children under 9 years
  3 or more cups for children 9 to 12 years
  4 cups or more for teenagers
  2 cups or more for adults
  3 cups or more for pregnant women
  4 cups or more for nursing mothers

Meat Group
  2 or more servings. Count as one serving:
    2 to 3 ounces lean, cooked beef, veal, pork, lamb, poultry,
      fish—without bone
    2 eggs
    1 cup cooked dry beans, dry peas, lentils
    4 tablespoons peanut butter

Vegetable-Fruit Group (½ cup serving, or 1 piece fruit, etc.)
  4 or more servings per day, including:
    1 serving of citrus fruit or other fruit or vegetable as a good
      source of vitamin C, or 2 servings of a fair source
    1 serving, at least every other day, of a dark-green or
      deep-yellow vegetable for vitamin A
    2 or more servings of other vegetables and fruits, including
      potatoes

Bread-Cereals Group
  4 or more servings daily (whole grain, enriched or restored).
    Count as one serving:
    1 slice bread
    1 ounce ready-to-eat cereal
    ½ to ¾ cup cooked cereal, corn meal, grits, macaroni,
      noodles, rice or spaghetti

SOURCE: U.S. Department of Agriculture, *"Consumers All* Yearbook of Agriculture, 1965," (Washington, D.C., 1965), p. 394

TABLE 12.2
DESIRABLE WEIGHTS FOR MEN AND WOMEN
According to Height and Frame, Ages 25 and Over

Height (in Shoes)*	Weight in Pounds (in Indoor Clothing)		
	Small Frame	Medium Frame	Large Frame
Men			
5' 2"	112–120	118–129	126–141
3"	115–123	121–133	129–144
4"	118–126	124–136	132–148
5"	121–129	127–139	135–152
6"	124–133	130–143	138–156
7"	128–137	134–147	142–161
8"	132–141	138–152	147–166
9"	136–145	142–156	151–170
10"	140–150	146–160	155–174
11"	144–154	150–165	159–179
6' 0"	148–158	154–170	164–184
1"	152–162	158–175	168–189
2"	156–167	162–180	173–194
3"	160–171	167–185	178–199
4"	164–175	172–190	182–204
Women			
4' 10"	92– 98	96–107	104–119
11"	94–101	98–110	106–122
5' 0"	96–104	101–113	109–125
1"	99–107	104–116	112–128
2"	102–110	107–119	115–131
3"	105–113	110–122	118–134
4"	108–116	113–126	121–138
5"	111–119	116–130	125–142
6"	114–123	120–135	129–146
7"	118–127	124–139	133–150
8"	122–131	128–143	137–154
9"	126–135	132–147	141–158
10"	130–140	136–151	145–163
11"	134–144	140–155	149–168
6' 0"	138–148	144–159	153–173

*1-inch heels for men and 2-inch heels for women.

SOURCE: Metopolitan Life Insurance Company. Derived primarily from data of the *Build and Blood Pressure Study, 1959*, Society of Actuaries. These figures are currently under revision.

pound of body fat therefore requires a reduction of 3,500 calories from your diet or the energy expenditure of 3,500 additional calories.

That means if you require 2,500 calories daily to maintain your ideal weight (at your present energy level), you could gain one pound each week (every seven days) simply by eating 500 more calories a day than you need. That's a weight increase of about four pounds a month or 48 pounds a year! On the other hand, by reversing the situation, you could also lose approximately four pounds a month or 48 pounds a year simply by reducing your intake by 500 calories per day or increasing your energy usage (activity level) enough to "burn off" 500 more calories per day.

The point is, however, whether you are trying to maintain your ideal weight or lose or gain weight, careful attention should be given to meeting your body's nutritional requirements. The best way to do this is by following the recommended plan of daily servings from each of the four basic food groups. Calories can be *wisely* added or subtracted by adjusting serving sizes. In this way, nutritional requirements can be met to better ensure good health, while caloric intake can be adjusted to match energy needs. It is important to note that a sound nutritional plan will provide you with all the nutrients your body requires, unless you have some special needs. (If so, you should be evaluated by a physician who can recommend the best nutritional plan to meet those unique needs.)

Many people take a multiple vitamin daily as a supplement to their nutritional plan—in a sense, as a means of insurance that all nutrient requirements have been met. Since so many foods are processed today, and because over-cooking can destroy nutrients, taking a daily supplemental vitamin/mineral tablet will usually do no harm and may be helpful for some people. The main point, though, is to balance your menu to meet at least the minimum daily requirements and add or subtract caloric intake according to your energy needs.

Nutrition for Certain Ages and Stages

The following is a discussion of some of the nutritional needs unique to certain stages in our lives. From infancy through the elderly years, nutrition plays a significant role in good health and well-being (or the lack of them). A general understanding of the special nutritional requirements at different ages and stages can help us better meet those needs.

Infancy

It is a well-established fact that the best food for a young infant is its mother's milk. It is produced in the right composition and the right amount for the baby, based on its sucking demands. In addition to its ideal composition of nutrients, mother's milk has certain other advantages: (1) There is less risk of a baby's developing allergies when it is not exposed to cow's milk or other proteins in early infancy; (2) human milk provides added resistance to infection, by passing on antibodies from the mother to the baby; and (3) there is little or no risk for iron deficiency anemia in the breast-fed infant.

Besides these benefits, breast-feeding allows a certain closeness and rapport to develop between the mother and baby. This "bonding" does not require nursing but may be easier to achieve with it. There is also a slightly reduced risk of obesity in the babies who are breast-fed in early infancy. For one thing, they tend not to be overfed and eat only what they want. Also, breast-fed infants are usually not given other foods until later in infancy.

When nursing is impossible or not preferred, commercially available infant formulas provide a nutritionally sound substitute for most infants. Cow's milk-based formulas have been modified by heating, removing certain ingredients of the cow's milk and adding other nutrients in order to be closest to "the perfect food" (mother's milk). They are relatively convenient and affordable and a better choice than home-prepared milks. Formulas contain vitamins and iron and can be given safely without added foods until 6 to 8 months of age.

When cow's milk-based formula is not tolerated by an infant or there is a strong allergy tendency in a family, a soy-based formula is usually recommended. Soy formulas are nutritious for babies and contain vitamins and iron, as well as the proper balance of protein, carbohydrates and fat for good growth. Other more specialized formulas are also available for babies with unique needs.

The question of when to introduce other foods besides breast milk or formula is often argued. While many babies have been fed "solid foods" even at several weeks of age and have done well with them, there is really no need to introduce solid foods before 3 to 4 months of age to formula-fed infants. Breast-fed infants do not need additional foods until at least 6 months of age. Some babies who receive foods early develop allergies, and many of them are obese as infants and children. (Fat babies tend to be more sick with respiratory infections than thin ones.)

When solid foods are introduced, common sense is the rule. Introduce one new food at a time, no oftener than once a week. If a baby does not seem to like a food, do not force it. Start with bland foods that are less likely to lead to allergy or stomach upset: cereal (rice, oatmeal or barley); white fruits (applesauce, pears, ripe bananas); yellow vegetables (squash, sweet potatoes, carrots). After several weeks of trying one new food at a time, a meat may be introduced (chicken, lamb, beef). Green vegetables and the "yellow" or colored fruits can be added later. (Babies do not seem to need variety—but parents do! Don't rush.)

Fruit juices and punches are really not needed for nutrition as long as a baby is taking breast milk or formula, but these are often given for variety. Remember that fruit juices and punches offer nearly as many calories as milk but less nutritional value. Babies can drink plain water (not sweetened) and will do so if they are thirsty. They will *learn* not to drink it, though, if they are always offered something sweet to drink.

Many families are choosing to prepare their own baby foods, which is quite a reasonable and healthy way to go. If you decide to make your own baby foods, take care not to add extra sugar or salt to foods. Do not over-cook foods, either, since over-cooking removes many valuable vitamins, minerals and nutrients. Babies can eat foods that contain some texture and small chunks, so don't over-grind or over-blend. They can eat certain foods right from the table—for example, mashed potatoes, mashed bananas, fork-mashed cottage cheese.

When babies start to put things in their mouths and chew on them—6 months and later—it is appropriate to give them something nutritious (but safe) to chew. While "teething biscuits" are traditional, they are messy and do not add much nourishment to the diet. Try a small piece of banana, a small piece of soft cheese, or a hard roll or bagel instead. A baby does not need teeth to be able to mouth these things. Always supervise a baby who is chewing on something—do not leave any infant or child unattended—in case choking should occur.

Cow's milk is not recommended until at least 6 months of age, but waiting until 1 year is even better. Unmodified cow's milk, if given early, is associated with not only milk allergy but also iron deficiency anemia. When it is introduced, whole milk is preferred, although 2 percent milk may be adequate for babies who are overweight. Skim milk is not a good food for infants for several reasons: It does not provide enough of the fats that babies need, and it contains too much protein and salt. When milk is introduced, it should be limited to 24 ounces a day, although 16 ounces is probably enough for a baby or child who is eating other foods.

Many parents ask about vitamins for their infants—and spend excessive amounts of money unnecessarily on such vitamins. Breast-fed infants probably do not need additional vitamins unless the mother is malnourished, but many doctors recommend A, C and D for the baby because of the potential risk of those vitamins' being inadequate in breast milk. Formula-fed infants receive the minimum requirement of vitamins in the formula and need no additional supplement if they drink close to a quart of formula in each 24-hour period.

Fluoride supplementation for infants and children has been very helpful in reducing the problem of dental decay. In areas where drinking water is not fluoridated, all babies should receive fluoride as prescribed by the doctor (do *not* exceed the dosage recommended). This can be given as drops or in combination with vitamins.

Iron is an important part of infant nutrition. All babies need iron in their diets during the first year. Breast-fed infants receive what they need through the milk until about 6 months but then need more dietary iron after that time. Meats and certain vegetables contain iron, and cereals are supplemented, although this iron may not be very usable. Formula-fed infants should receive formula that contains iron during the first year of life. (This does not produce increased gas or stomach upset, contrary to what people think.)

Parents should not worry about their baby's nutritional needs as long as these basic guidelines are followed. In fact, it is really very easy to meet all of the infant's nutritional needs. It is through a combination of basic principles and common sense, backed up by sound advice from the doctor when questions arise, that parents can feel confident of their ability to provide good nutrition for their baby.

Childhood

When babies are about a year old, their growth slows down, and they need less food for their weight than they did even a few months earlier. About the same time, they also become more independent, saying to the world, in essence, "I'd rather do it myself." This extends into feeding, and they want to feed themselves, no matter how clumsily. They may also refuse to eat only because of being stubborn—and show more discrimination about *what* they eat as well as when. At this stage many food battles begin, often to continue into adolescence and adulthood. And many bad eating habits are started—often innocently.

Trying to have a baby eat a balanced, healthy diet at this stage can be exasperating. Many parents are frustrated because the baby (and later the child) won't eat what is put on the table—or won't eat "enough to keep a bird alive." Others fall into the snacking trap—thinking the child is not eating enough.

Children, like adults, need foods from each of the basic four food groups every day. Most children actually like foods from all these groups and will happily eat them—as long as no force is applied and care is used in how they are presented. One or more servings from each group every day is all that's important—the order or "menu" doesn't matter.

There are several pitfalls in feeding children that, if avoided, can lead to happier mealtimes and healthier diets. One is the tendency to allow children to "drink" their meals. They drink too much milk or too much juice or too much soda, then have no appetite for food because they have already taken in most of their caloric requirement. Limit milk drinking to 16 ounces a day in the first five to six years, to 24 ounces (three glasses) until adolescence and to one quart after adolescence. Encourage children to drink water if they are thirsty and limit sweet drinks, including juices and punches, severely. (Punches are not nutritious and contribute to obesity and dental decay.)

Another pitfall is assuming a child is not eating enough—either because of what you see the child eat, or because he or she looks "skinny." The result may be nagging—and the child's response of "picking." Set limits for the time of meals, then remove the food and offer *no* snacks until the next meal. This includes juice, milk and other liquids. (A child will not starve, even if he or she does not eat for several days.)

An even more common situation occurs when a child is assumed to eat very little, but when you really assess the situation, he or she is eating quite well—by snacking. Dry cereal in the morning, a glass of milk at mid-morning, part of a sandwich and a cookie for lunch, a piece of fruit after school, a few bites of dinner, then ice cream before bedtime actually turns out to be quite a bit of food—but not eaten at mealtimes.

Certain children are, by nature, picky eaters. They are fussy about what they eat and when they eat it. They do not like variety, preferring to eat a peanut butter sandwich three times a day for months. These children are frustrating but often very healthy. They eat when they are hungry, not when others want them to. Do not fall into the trap of fixing special treats because the child "will starve to death." Offer very small portions and allow the child to ask for more if he or she wants more. Looking at a heaping plate if you're not hungry is overwhelming.

So-called "junk foods" and "fast foods" have become a problem for many children and many families. Avoid them as snacks and stock the house with nutritious snack foods: raisins fruit, nuts (for children over 3 or so), whole-grain snacks and granola, cheese, yogurt. Limit sweets sharply, offering instead the fruits and yogurt. Limit "fast foods" to an occasional, not routine, item on the menu (even though not all "fast foods" are all bad).

There is a possibility that a sensible diet in childhood can prevent certain of the problems of aging: cardiovascular disease, obesity and others. Many suggest that limiting the amount of fat in the diet, limiting egg intake to three or four a week, and avoiding salt and food additives will be preventive. The answers are not all in, but such limits will certainly teach a child solid eating habits for the future—part of any parent's goal.

Adolescence

Adolescence is a time of rapid growth, with a need for increased food intake, enough to build sound, healthy bodies. Unfortunately, it is also a time when youngsters are likely to eat erratically and be somewhat out of the control of their parents. This presents a dilemma as to how to best meet a developing youngster's nutritional needs.

Ideally, the best nutritional plan during adolescence is a well-balanced diet that includes selections from the four basic food groups, without emphasis on any one food substance. A slightly increased proportion of protein may be useful but is not essential. This nutritional plan can be met by foods the adolescent—and his or her friends—will eat, but it requires creativity and an approach that does not cause rebellion.

"Fast foods" and "junk foods" are a concern with the adolescent. The peer pressure to eat with the gang at the local hangout is great, even when youngsters have had a strong foundation in nutritional principles at home. Not all fast foods are junk, and as long as there is some balance between carbohydrates, fat and protein, the diet can be relatively sound. The potential trouble can arise when the youngster eats an abundance of sweets and carbohydrates, without protein. This adds calories but in less-than-perfect foods. Try to balance this pattern by making good, nutritious snacks available at home and preparing nutritionally balanced but appealing meals at home. Try to encourage a youngster to start the day with a well-balanced breakfast. Engourage the drinking of milk (a quart a day is enough) and juices rather than sodas.

Many adolescent girls are very concerned about excess weight. They "watch their weight," following unusual fad diets that their friends have heard about. They usually lose a few pounds, only to regain them when there is a special event, or they simply abandon the fad diet because they tire of it. Many times the adolescent has a misguided idea about what is "fattening" and what is not—and eats far more calories in an attempt to lose weight than would have happened if she had stuck to her regular diet.

Most of the "dieting" that adolescent girls do is not overly dangerous, although not particularly healthy. Be aware, however, of the danger signs for anorexia nervosa (a very serious eating disorder): excessive weight loss to the point of emaciation; refusal to eat at all or refusal to eat anything except a bizarre assortment of foods; vomiting after eating a large meal; and changes in body image that make a girl see herself as "fat" while being, in fact, starved. This problem or potential problem requires intensive medical and psychiatric care.

Of some concern are the young girls who become pregnant while teen-agers. These youngsters are often poorly nourished before pregnancy, then "diet" in an attempt to cover the weight gain of pregnancy. They are at particular risk for problems, both for themselves and their unborn babies. Ideally, sound nutritional habits prior to pregnancy will protect against some of the danger. And girls who are pregnant as adolescents have a special need for a sound diet—not only in order to protect their developing baby and its growth but to assure their own growth and development.

Teen-agers who are already overweight have a particular problem during adolescence, when appetite is often large, and social pressures are great to eat what the others are eating. It is very difficult for a fat teen-ager to lose weight, but it may be possible for him or her *not to gain*, while continuing to grow in height. This is often realistic as a goal, with the success rate much greater than that for an actual weight-reduction program. It can be done by limiting the quantity of food eaten and avoiding the obviously fattening "empty" carbohydrates. A very important aspect of weight control for these and other adolescents is activity—just moving rather than sitting will help.

For adolescents who are motivated to lose weight, a sensible plan that stresses good eating habits for the future and a slow, steady weight loss is best. It is important that dietary restrictions not be excessive, so muscle and bone tissue is not sacrificed during the rapid-growth period. Again, a well-balanced plan that allows for some personal freedom and the ability to "be like the others" is most likely to succeed. Nagging and pressure by parents are usually met by natural rebellion.

Adolescents, whether male or female, who are athletes have special needs that are discussed later in this chapter (see "The Athlete"). However, here again, attempts to gain or lose weight rapidly are common and not healthy. The best approach to either gaining or losing weight is a sound, balanced nutritional plan.

Many teen-agers are concerned, whether for short or long periods of time, about eating meat—and become vegetarians. Parents not familiar with vegetarian diets become concerned, unnecessarily. (Most youngsters eliminate only red meats on this kind of diet, and many do so temporarily.) A vegetarian diet can be very sound nutritionally, and many believe it is more healthy than a diet containing meat. As long as the youngster eats food that contains a balance of vegetable proteins and also drinks milk and eats eggs, the diet is probably healthy. If fish is also eaten, all the nutritional needs are easily met.

The concerns many parents have about their teen-agers' nutrition are frequently justified, and it is often possible to intervene constructively to improve the situation. This should be done creatively, without force, so the teen-ager is more likely to comply. Also, good, sound nutritional principles (which have been learned in the family prior to adolescence) will aid the youngster in choosing foods that are healthy for growth and energy. Fortunately, there is great emphasis on health and fitness these days—a factor that makes more adolescents conscious of the importance of proper weight and nutritional health.

Adulthood

There really are no dietary guidelines unique to the adult, other than following a well-balanced and healthy nutritional plan, using the four food groups as the foundation for planning menus and taking care to avoid overindulgence. Unless someone has maintained a high activity level into adulthood, often fewer calories are necessary to meet energy needs. If caloric intake is not reduced to match the reduction in calorie use, slowly but surely (and sometimes rapidly), weight will be gained.

You may have heard someone say, "I just don't understand it! I'm eating the same as I did a few years ago, but I'm gaining weight." What occurs in many adults is slow weight gain, but it all adds up. Just think, if you eat only a little more food (or reduce your activity level but not your caloric intake) to gain just 4 pounds a year—in five years you will be 20 pounds overweight. That's what people mean when they say weight sneaks up on them!

One remedy is to weigh yourself routinely. If in one week's time you experience a gain of 2 pounds, reduce your caloric intake for the next seven days and get rid of those 2 pounds before they become permanent and you get used to that extra "little" weight. This can simply snowball on you, and before you know it, you are 10, 20, 30, 40 or even 50 pounds overweight!

Although a well-balanced nutritional plan (with care taken about the number of calories consumed per day) is the best means of assuring proper fuel for the adult body, there are a few other principles you might consider applying to your nutritional plan. Recent research points to lowered risk for hypertension, heart disease and some cancers if these principles become part of your dietary regimen:

- Emphasize fiber intake in the diet.
- Emphasize a low-fat intake, especially of saturated fats found in animal meats, butter and some cheeses. When fats are eaten, try to use polyunsaturated vegetable fats, but sparingly.
- Emphasize a low-sodium (salt) intake. One of the best ways to reduce salt intake is to salt lightly while cooking but *never* put a saltshaker on the table. Get accustomed to other seasonings.

Most adults often eat too much of the wrong foods—instead of simply eating too much. Both exercise and proper diet are vital to ensure a healthy life as we age. Care should be taken to follow a well-balanced nutritional plan that will provide our bodies with all the vitamins, minerals, proteins, fats and carbohydrates they need for continued cell production as well as the energy we need for overall good health and a long life.

Old Age

We often forget that as we grow older (most particularly past 60 years of age), we need to pay more attention to our nutritional status—not less. It is actually a fallacy (and indeed a very damaging one) that we need no longer be concerned about what we eat once we are older. If anything, the opposite is true! In fact, good nutrition plays a significant role in better health and feeling well as we grow older.

Poor nutrition among the elderly is at an epidemic level. It is a serious public health concern. Often those who are advanced in years are unaware of the importance good nutrition has for them (or those who care for someone elderly have little or no concept of the nutritional needs and unique problems of the elderly). After the age of 59, there appear to be more deficiencies in protein, calcium, iron and vitamin A, as well as many reported deficiencies in ascorbic acid, folic acid, vitamin D and serum albumin (one of the proteins).

Ironically, even though poor nutrition is epidemic among the elderly, so is obesity. Obesity is implicated as a contributing factor in many serious illnesses or health problems. It also puts more stress on the heart and circulatory system, other organs and the joints.

There are essentially three areas where the older person can make a difference in his or her own health: by staying physically fit (through some form of exercise); by maintaining ideal weight; and by following proper nutritional guidelines.

There are, however, many problems relatively unique to the elderly that make good nutritional habits more difficult. Some of these include:

- A decrease in metabolism.
- Poor appetite.
- Difficulty chewing food because of poor teeth or ill-fitting dentures.
- Sometimes swallowing difficulty.
- Decrease in physical activity (either by choice or as a result of arthritis, bursitis, stiffness or other problems).
- A decrease (or changes) in the ability to taste, smell or see (all important to appetite).
- The onset of frequent illnesses, chronic disease or pain as a result of disease, illness or injury.
- Constipation (which makes many people lose their desire to eat).

- The use of many medications (because of more health problems or aches and pains) and the use of alcohol (both of which tend to reduce appetite substantially).
- Senility (degrees of mental deterioration).
- Depression.
- Loneliness or isolation.
- Poverty.

Some of these problems have no easy answers. Others can be remedied by education, by medical intervention and sometimes (most importantly) by someone who cares about the elderly person's health and well-being.

A sound diet for an older person should most often be high in protein, vitamins and minerals. (Those with a chronic illness, such as diabetes or heart disease, need to follow a nutritional plan prescribed by their doctor.) Emphasis should be placed on meeting the minimum daily requirements for nutrients, with special care to ensure an adequate amount of protein, calcium, vitamin A, ascorbic acid, folic acid and vitamin D. Milk products—such as milk, cheese, cottage cheese and yogurt—are important, as are proteins found in meats, fish, poultry, veal, pork and eggs.

If requirements (number of servings) are met daily, then calcium and iron deficiencies can more than likely be avoided. Iron deficiency can result in anemia (and a feeling of overall weakness). Calcium deficiency can result in "soft" bones (osteoporosis) and therefore many broken bones. Menopausal and postmenopausal women must be especially careful to supplement their calcium intake to avoid osteoporosis. Women also tend to have more need for iron supplementation than men (although both should take note of this requirement as they age).

If meats (and other proteins) are difficult to chew or swallow, they can be stewed or even blended and made into soup. Chopped or blended meats, fish and poultry make good sandwich spreads as well. A diet high in fiber (fruits, vegetables, whole grains, bran, etc.) will also aid in reducing the incidence of constipation and provide vital vitamins, minerals and carbohydrates. Fluid intake, particularly water, is important and should be emphasized. However, fruit juices and other beverages also help meet fluid needs. Many smaller meals throughout the day (instead of three larger meals) aid in digestion and may encourage the older person to eat. A little of this and a little of that is easier to take (and digest) than a huge meal that immediately turns the person away. Taking a daily multiple vitamin with iron is usually a good idea as well.

It's important to remember that nutritional deficiencies work in a vicious circle. If the person is not getting enough iron and anemia occurs, he or she feels "too weak to eat" or is simply "not hungry." If a calcium deficiency results in brittle bones and a fall breaks a hip or other bone, then there is pain and loss of appetite, and the person becomes less active (which can result in depression, greater loss of appetite and even constipation, when he or she does eat). Therefore, the best way to avoid all the potential complications is to prevent the nutritional deficiencies from occurring. People simply feel better, do better and are more active when eating properly.

Those who care for or care about an older person should encourage proper nutrition, make food easy to eat and appealing and allow the older person to enjoy more of the foods he or she particularly likes (as long as all other nutritional requirements are being met and the foods are not restricted because of the need for a special diet). If someone wants a tuna sandwich for lunch every day, that's fine. Maybe you can encourage him or her to have a glass of milk and a small salad or vegetable with it. What you should be concerned with is that all nutritional requirements are met. If someone likes to eat the same foods every day, and these meet all nutritional requirements, there is no need to enforce variety on the person. If he or she doesn't seem to like anything, then try offering a variety of choices, change the type or increase the use of spices, and see if you can find foods that the person will eat that also match nutritional requirements.

Watch calories with those who eat fattening foods out of frustration, loneliness or for gratification. They can become tremendously overweight very rapidly, and this can endanger their health. Encouraging long walks (for those who are able) helps burn off calories and will make them feel better.

Those with Very Special Needs

As we have already discussed in this chapter, at certain stages in our lives (infancy, childhood, adulthood and in our elderly years), we have unique nutritional needs. But beyond these, there are many other situations that demand either temporary or continual very special nutritional measures.

The woman who is pregnant or trying to get pregnant, the nursing mother and the athlete have additional nutrient and/or energy requirements. Those with a chronic health problem—such as diabetes, cardiovascular disease or hypertension, and cancer—

also have very special nutritional needs. And the overweight or obese person is facing a unique health problem where nutrition plays a starring role.

In the following section we will discuss some of the situations where nutritional guidance and specific dietary plans are essential. For those who have such unique nutritional needs, their personal physician, often in conjunction with a registered dietitian, will of course recommend the specific nutritional program best suited for them. However, the following basic information gives a general overview of some of the dietary programs and problems faced by those with very special nutritional requirements.

The Pregnant Woman

Much has been said and written over the years about nutrition and pregnancy, and much has been misunderstood. Old wives' tales abound, as do numerous evangelical advocates for one "miracle" nutritional plan after another. Most often, these miracle plans are not based on medical fact, which is the very reason you find hundreds of such diets claiming to be the best for the pregnant woman. Each new dietary fad promises to deliver the healthiest baby in the world.

The reason so much conflict can exist is that all the answers about diet and pregnancy are not known. While medical science now has a great many answers, many questions or gray areas still remain. This leaves the situation wide open and often places the expectant mother at the mercy of what she or others have heard about "the diet" to follow during pregnancy.

Certainly no one questions the importance of special nutritional needs during pregnancy. But "special" in this case means following a nutritional plan that promotes good health and safety during pregnancy, not some exotic concoction or specific foods to be consumed each day of the week or during certain stages of pregnancy.

In actuality, the diet for the expectant mother is based on simple, reasonable, sound and basic nutritional principles. Most experts agree that the nine months of pregnancy are vital times for building the human edifice—with cells multiplying and dividing rapidly and organs and body systems forming and developing.

Each of us has a choice about what we will or will not eat, how often and how much we will eat, and how reasonable our eating habits will be. We decide if we will follow a constructive, well-planned diet or not. The unborn baby does not have this luxury of choices. Only the expectant mother can control what the unborn baby will "eat"—only she can control the "diet" of the rapidly growing and developing little being. It is therefore essential that she understand the basic nutritional principles and guidelines to follow during pregnancy.

First of all, a well-balanced diet during pregnancy is best, not only for the unborn baby but also for the expectant mother. A balanced nutritional plan involves the following:

- Using the four basic food groups as a general guide and eating recommended portions every day. The number and size of servings from each food group and those foods your doctor may emphasize more than others will depend on your own nutritional needs and any necessary dietary restrictions you may have during pregnancy. By having specific servings from the four food groups daily, you can be assured that you and your unborn baby are receiving a balance of proteins, carbohydrates and fats, as well as essential vitamins and minerals.
- Eating enough calories to gain between 20 and 30 pounds during the nine months of pregnancy, with most of this gain occurring during the last six months.
- Having enough iron in your diet to maintain your own good health and that of the unborn baby. Many doctors recommend and prescribe iron supplements or vitamins including iron to ensure that there is enough iron available for extra blood production during pregnancy.

A few precautionary notes:

1. Pregnancy is not the time to go on a weight-reduction diet. Restriction of carbohydrates (starches and sugars) in particular can be dangerous to the unborn baby. Recent studies show that carbohydrate restriction may result in a greater incidence of babies with lower intelligence levels and physical underdevelopment. Women who gain less than 10 pounds during pregnancy are at serious risk for stillbirth, premature birth and having a baby who is undergrown and not fully developed. However, this is not to say more carbohydrates are better. Rather, your emphasis should be on meeting the minimum daily requirements of carbohydrates for optimal health and safety for both you and your unborn baby.
2. Megavitamins are vitamins packaged or taken in large doses—and they are drugs. Vitamins or supplements not

prescribed by your doctor should not be taken, and no one should take more than the amount prescribed or recommended. Again, more is not better. If you are following a sound nutritional plan, you are meeting the needs of pregnancy. Vitamins and supplements are usually prescribed as "insurance," to guarantee that the baby does not experience any vitamin deficiencies. If certain vitamins and minerals are not in an expectant mother's diet, certain maternal deficiencies occur. If vitamins, minerals and supplements are taken as prescribed, they will not harm the mother or the unborn baby. However, excesses may be harmful and should be avoided.

3. Needing extra protein in the diet during pregnancy is another fallacy. Research has shown that a pregnant woman only needs to consume a normal daily requirement of protein. If a woman prefers a higher protein intake and her physician feels this is not contraindicated (she can afford the extra calories), then this additional amount of protein will cause no harm. It is important to remember, however, that carbohydrate consumption (meeting the daily requirement) is vital and has proved to be more important than protein consumption.

In situations where there is too much weight gain during pregnancy (fat is being put on), it is often due to eating more than your necessary daily requirements of carbohydrates, fats and proteins. Basically, the serving sizes are too large. A workable solution can usually be found if you and your doctor go over what foods and serving sizes you have been eating and adjust food servings accordingly. Being overweight during pregnancy is not healthy either and puts more stress on the cardiovascular system. Care should be taken to eat properly and meet all nutritional requirements for good health and safety but not overindulge (adding useless fat to the body) during the nine months of pregnancy.

For women who are already overweight, it is always best to lose excess pounds *before* getting pregnant. (Losing excess weight does make a difference—the baby's weight correlates with your weight before pregnancy: Overweight women tend to have large babies.) No one should start a reducing diet once pregnant or while trying to get pregnant.

Often, though, a woman will not even know she has conceived until two or three months into a pregnancy. Yet those first three months are vital for fetal cell and organ development.

Therefore, if you're planning for a child, also plan your nutritional needs and make sure they are met while you are trying to get pregnant. This "pre-pregnancy" period, then, is the ideal time to begin a sound, well-balanced nutritional program. Discuss the best dietary plan for you with your doctor ahead of time and be sure to ask plenty of questions so you feel sure you understand the dos and don'ts. This is of particular importance to women who have special dietary requirements due to a chronic condition such as diabetes, heart disease, hypertension and others.

The Nursing Mother

Nursing a baby requires a well-planned and balanced nutritional regimen for the mother—in order that both she and her baby do well. There are many myths about what a nursing mother should and should not eat. These often frighten the nursing mother unnecessarily. As with many other special conditions, a sound, commonsense approach is best.

Human milk is produced by converting "fuel"—food taken in by the mother—into a food source for the baby. This production of food requires additional food in the mother's diet, even more than was needed during pregnancy. Just after birth and for the baby's first few months, the mother needs an additional 400 to 600 calories of energy a day to produce milk, and this increases to 600 to 800 calories as the baby grows. These calories should be provided by selecting foods from the four basic food groups, with about one-third to one-half of them coming from a protein source. Eat an extra serving of meat, fish or eggs, and drink about one quart of milk a day. Additional milk protein may be taken as cheese, yogurt or ice cream (but don't overdo!).

One of the most important aspects of producing sufficient breast milk is drinking enough liquids to make the volume of milk needed. Drink at least three quarts of liquids a day, with at least two quarts being something other than milk (fruit juices and water are good choices, with soft drinks being less nutritious). Try to drink a glass of liquid each time you nurse as a means of remembering to drink enough. Avoid coffee, tea and cola drinks, because their caffeine content can make the baby jittery and fussy.

Nursing mothers need to continue the vitamin supplements that they were given during pregnancy. They should also make sure they have adequate iron intake (either in the diet or with the addition of iron supplements recommended by the doctor). Added protein or other supplements are normally not needed unless the doctor has determined that the mother herself has increased demands for nutrients.

There are many beliefs about foods to avoid while nursing, many of which are myths that place unnecessary restrictions and worries on mothers. While it is true that certain babies seem to have gas when their mothers eat certain foods, common sense should prevail—avoid *excesses* of anything. If the baby has a fussy period, look back at what you had eaten at the previous two meals and make a mental note of it. If fussiness occurs again and you had eaten something similar, perhaps you might want to avoid that food (or foods) in the future. Some babies have touchier stomachs than others and may react to the "gassy" foods—cabbage relatives, onions, garlic and spices. Chocolate contains a substance similar to caffeine, and excessive intake may cause fussiness. Again, avoid excesses.

As is true with other conditions that increase the body's needs for nutrition, nursing places extra demands on the mother, whose health will suffer if her diet is inadequate. Here, too, common sense and a well-balanced nutritional plan with foods taken from the four food groups are the rules.

The Athlete

Many dietary plans have been touted as being "the best" for athletic performance and physical fitness. But the nutritional requirements of the athlete are easy to meet and do not necessarily include specialized foods, nutrients or supplements. Years of research into the effects of various diets on performance show that there is no "miracle diet." A well-balanced nutritional plan that is based on the four food groups will supply the athlete with necessary energy and fuel.

In most cases the only special requirements for those involved in strenuous activities and conditioning regimens will be greater total food intake to meet the body's increased energy needs. The more exercise a person gets, the more fuel is needed to expend more energy. As energy needs increase, more calories will be needed (unless weight reduction is the goal). Increasing the serving sizes but still following a well-balanced nutritional plan is always best.

A well-balanced, healthful diet is capable of supplying all the energy an athlete needs. The use of vitamin supplements, megavitamins, minerals, additional protein or amino acids is unnecessary unless the person has a specific deficiency that his or her doctor has identified and for which a supplement has been prescribed. Basically, use of supplements is not known to improve performance—and is a waste of money for the athlete.

Some vitamins or minerals or combinations taken in large quantities can be quite dangerous. Excessive doses of vitamin B complex will be eliminated by the body, but niacin (nicotinic acid) may cause damage to the heart muscle with strenuous activity. Vitamins A and D, as well as iron, can jeopardize the athlete's health if taken to excess. A daily multivitamin will do no harm as a supplement, but even this is unnecessary for a person who is following a well-planned nutritional regimen.

Rapid weight gain or weight reduction to qualify for competition is not healthy. When weight (and muscles) need to be built, it is best done gradually. Use of drugs to stimulate or suppress appetite is to be condemned as a potentially dangerous, life-threatening practice.

There has been much argument about what an athlete should eat before a competition or large burst of activity. A well-balanced meal, perhaps higher in carbohydrates than usual, eaten about two to three hours before activity is usually best tolerated and provides the athlete with enough fuel to compete, while not slowing him or her down. It is vital that there always be enough water or other liquid to drink freely to prevent dehydration because of sweating. While the athlete needs enough salt in the diet to produce sweat, excess salt intake in the form of salt tablets is not recommended.

The picture for the athlete when it comes to nutrition is the same as for most others: a well-balanced diet, sensible in what it contains—with enough calories and nutrients to meet that specific active person's energy requirements. Extreme variation from the usual dietary plan is unnecessary and potentially dangerous.

The Diabetic

Diabetes (diabetes mellitus) is a disease caused by either a deficiency in insulin production or inefficient insulin action. This leads to several problems: (1) the inability of the body to use sugar (glucose) for energy and cellular functions and a consequent buildup of glucose in the blood (hyperglycemia) and (2) an increased breakdown of body fat in an attempt to use it for energy. The fat breakdown is inefficient and leads to a buildup of ketones in the blood ("ketosis"). When metabolism becomes very inefficient, acid also builds up in the blood and tissues ("acidosis"). When this "ketoacidosis" occurs, it is a potentially life-threatening process because of the buildup of abnormal products that poison the body's cells.

There are two different kinds of diabetes mellitus—*insulin dependent* and *non-insulin dependent*. Insulin-dependent diabetes cannot be prevented or cured—but it can be controlled. It requires the daily injection of insulin into the body, along with a careful dietary regimen. It often occurs in childhood but can start later in life as well.

Non-insulin-dependent diabetes is usually a disease of adulthood and is a result of obesity about 70 percent of the time. In this form of diabetes, insulin is actually produced by the pancreas, sometimes in even more than normal amounts, but the insulin is inefficiently used in the body. Weight loss (to one's ideal, healthy weight) most often results in a return to normal breakdown and use of the blood sugar for energy.

With the development of insulin in 1922, it was hoped that the answer had finally been found for the diabetic. The development and availability of insulin injections were major breakthroughs and have saved countless lives. But it became clear that insulin was only part of the answer—and then only for some diabetics.

There are many vital aspects to managing either kind of diabetes. A controlled diet, regular exercise, stress control, weight control and insulin dosage (for insulin-dependent diabetics) are all important. Without each of these, diabetes may be poorly controlled and its complications more likely to develop.

The fact is, diet is one of the most important factors in the control of diabetes. It is much more complicated than simply "sort of" eating correctly. Following a balanced and specific nutritional plan must become a way of life for the diabetic. This nutritional plan is based on many different variables (height, ideal weight, body type and build, age, sex, whether weight loss is necessary or not, the amount of exercise regularly performed, overall energy demands and insulin dosage, as indicated).

Because of the complexity of determining the right nutritional plan for each individual based on these many factors, it is impossible to discuss the diabetic diet other than in general terms. The point is, the diabetic diet must be individualized for each diabetic. Usually, the person's physician and a registered dietitian reach what is essentially a "nutritional prescription" for that person and his or her specific needs. This takes time and careful evaluation. It also requires an educational process to ensure that the diabetic understands the diet prescription and is committed to following it. Presented below, then, are the broad dietary guidelines that most often apply to diabetes.

The first step in diabetes control is to try to allow the body to use rather than waste glucose. For insulin-dependent diabetics, this involves administration (by injection) of insulin and adjustment of their diet. For non-insulin-dependent diabetics, this requires careful adjustment of the diet. For both it requires a nutritional plan that allows the diabetic to reach his or her ideal weight. For the obese, non-insulin-dependent diabetic, this usually means weight reduction, and for some insulin-dependent persons, it means weight gain. After the ideal weight has been reached, the nutritional prescription is adjusted to meet the person's energy needs while still maintaining the ideal weight.

The diabetic nutritional plan is composed of 50 percent carbohydrate, 30 percent fat and 20 percent protein. The diet is also low in cholesterol, trigylcerides, salt and saturated fats, as a preventive measure against arteriosclerosis, coronary artery disease, hypertension and other heart and vascular problems for which the diabetic is at high risk.

The "exchange system" is most often used for prescribing the diabetic nutritional plan. The system was developed and is routinely revised by the American Dietetic Association, the American Diabetes Association Inc. and the U.S. Public Health Service's (Department of Health and Human Resources) Chronic Disease Program.

The exchange system plan is easy to use once it is understood. Foods are grouped based on their composition (fat, protein, carbohydrate) and their food value. Those in the same group have about the same composition and food value and can therefore be "exchanged" as long as the serving size indicated is followed carefully. Thus the plan, while controlling the value and composition of foods, also allows for variety, personal choice and ease in determining menus.

The plan is broken down into six exchange groups: (1) milk, (2) vegetable, (3) fruit, (4) bread, (5) meat and (6) fat exchanges. The number of choices (exchanges) allowed from each group each day is individualized, based on the physician's and dietitian's nutritional prescription. Dinner might include (as an example only): an exchange from the milk-exchange list, two exchanges from the fruit group, two vegetable exchanges, one exchange from the bread group, one meat exchange and one fat exchange. From the fruit exchanges, you might choose 1/2 cup of blackberries or 2 medium apricots or 17 small cherries or 1/2 cup of orange juice (or many others). Note that although the *amount* which can be eaten of a choice changes, the decision about *what* to have is yours.

Young children and teen-agers with diabetes can be a problem when it comes to diet. Many of them do not eat regularly and cannot be forced to do so. They are sometimes picky and don't always get hungry at the same times of the day. For this reason, their dietary management can be tricky.

Some diabetic children are managed with the exchange system, while others use the "TAG system," in which foods are selected based on "*total available glucose*" in the food. This assigns a number value to a food, allowing a parent or child to calculate roughly how much glucose needs to be covered by insulin. (Remember, diabetic children have the insulin-dependent form of diabetes.) It's just another way of looking at food—the balance of the diet and the number of calories are the same in either system. This diet, too, requires several educational sessions to learn. It may allow children and adolescents a bit more freedom to be more like their peers.

In general, the goal of treatment of diabetes for both adults and children is to keep their blood sugar relatively stable and near the normal range. This is done partly by dividing the food intake during the day into several small meals—usually three meals and three snacks. Following their nutritional prescription is important so that wide swings in blood sugar do not occur and proper foods are consumed. The pattern of the meals is usually adjusted on an individual basis, in order to fit in as much as possible with a person's usual habits and life-style, while still reaching the goal of stabilizing the blood sugar. By carefully following the nutritional prescription designed for them, both adults and children with diabetes can best control the disease and live happier and healthier lives.

The Person with Cardiovascular Disease or Hypertension

Unfortunately, the nutritional plan for the person with cardiovascular disease depends entirely on the type of problem. This makes it very difficult to generalize. However, certain basic premises can be outlined for those with hypertension and others with cardiovascular disease:

- The nutritional plan is usually designed to take off excess weight, which reduces the demand placed on the heart. Usually the goal is to keep heart patients slightly on the lean side.
- Six small meals throughout the day are often recommended over the traditional three large meals. Bulky, large meals put pressure on the heart and require greater cardiac output.

- Stimulants such as caffeine-containing drinks or foods are usually limited.
- Emphasis is generally placed on lowering the cholesterol level in the blood by means of a diet low in both saturated fats and cholesterol.
- Emphasis is usually placed on some degree of sodium (salt) restriction. The extent of sodium restriction will depend on the particular problem and its severity.
- In general, diets are low in animal fats and protein and a little higher in carbohydrates (with carbohydrates representing about 50 percent of total calories).
- Some diets for those who are hypertensive emphasize high fiber intake as well.

Diet is usually only part of the new regimen for the person with cardiovascular disease or hypertension. Exercise, the control of stress, adequate rest and relaxation, proper use of prescribed medications, stopping smoking (if the person smokes tobacco) and reduction in the use of alcohol are all part of a new life-style, along with the special nutritional plan.

The goals of diets for cardiovascular disease and hypertension are to avoid (or decrease the impact of) atherosclerosis (narrowing in the walls of the blood vessels); avoid putting any unnecessary stress on the heart; reduce the body's basal metabolism (metabolic rate at rest); prevent edema (fluid retention); and reduce blood pressure to normal or to the low-normal range.

The Person with Cancer

When it comes to nutrition, the greatest problems most people with cancer face are lack of appetite and, consequently, a lack of adequate caloric intake. Often cancer therapy causes constant upset stomach or nausea; vomiting when food is eaten or even when liquids are taken; changes in how things taste (they often taste quite bitter and unappetizing); stomatitis (inflammation of the mouth); which makes it painful to even put food into the mouth and chew; swallowing problems with some cancers (and their treatment), which make eating difficult or painful; and problems with malabsorption, which means that more calories (food) must be consumed in order to meet nutritional needs (and this is often difficult if side effects such as vomiting and nausea are occurring).

However, some recent research shows that adequate nutrition may have a positive effect on cancer therapy. Many people seem to tolerate chemotherapy better; their immune system appears to work more efficiently; at times the interval between chemotherapeutic dosages can be reduced; and if they can keep food down, they tend to feel better and stronger. Keeping one's nutritional status up may also have a positive effect on the tumor response, while malnutrition may result in a poorer response.

It is often helpful for the person with cancer to try many types of foods and liquids to see which ones he or she can tolerate best. There should always be an attempt to follow a well-balanced nutritional plan, but at times this is not realistic, and emphasis must be placed on caloric intake and consuming food choices that are best tolerated. Additional dietary support can be achieved by liquid nutritional formulas. Many commercially prepared liquid formulas or powdered preparations are presently available that can be added to milk or to another liquid. The person's physician may recommend one or have the cancer patient try many until he or she finds the one best tolerated or liked. Other people prefer to eat foods that are high in energy and calories instead of drinking the liquid supplements.

When necessary, the liquid supplements are the sole source of nutrition (unless intravenous feeding is also employed, but this is done in the hospital in most cases). If the mouth is inflamed (stomatitis) and food causes severe pain in the mouth, the liquid formulas are often used. Some people also make slushes or popsicles out of fruit juices. These are not only a good source of calorie intake and high in carbohydrates (which produce energy for the body), but the coldness feels good on the gums, tongue and mouth tissues. Popsicles can be made in commercially available popsicle molds or simply by putting a popsicle stick in the center of each cube of an ice cube tray. Slushes are also easy to make. The fruit juice is frozen in ice cube trays, then the cubes are thrown into a blender to "slush" them. Here's another possibility to consider: Some people may find that cold foods cause less nausea and vomiting than heated foods. Having many smaller meals throughout the day instead of three larger meals is often helpful. Also, some people seem to do quite well at breakfast and less well at subsequent meals. If this is the case, eating as much as possible at breakfast may help make up for the other meals where food is less well tolerated.

The point is, the ideal goal for the cancer patient is to eat as much as possible and support food intake by liquid nutritional formulas. By keeping his or her energy level up (done by meeting nutritional needs) the person with cancer usually feels better and may even do better.

To accomplish this requires a real commitment on the part of the cancer patient and those around him or her. It takes a concerted effort on everyone's part to ensure that nutritional needs are met. Patience and understanding are also important for family and friends of someone with cancer. It is never easy to eat when you are nauseated or constantly vomiting. Encouragement is helpful—making meeting nutritional needs a family effort—but anger and threats will often only make things worse. It is vital that everyone understand how valuable good nutrition is in helping the person fight the cancer.

The Overweight or Obese Person

Even with the current interest in and preoccupation with weight and good looks, the great majority of Americans are over-nourished, overweight or definitely obese. The fact that so many people are on weight-reduction programs and there are so many "miracle diets" is indication enough of the widespread nature of the problem and the difficulty people have in dealing with it.

The soundest weight-reduction program is one that is well planned and includes:

- A reduction in food intake to below that of the body's requirements for the day.
- An exercise and activity regimen that increases the body's expenditure of energy.
- Modification of eating habits toward the development of a new and healthier life-style (in essence, a diet should be *permanent*, not temporary).
- Work on attitude, self-image and self-concept.

Most sensible diets have as a goal a weight loss of about two pounds a week after the first week (when loss is often larger). They involve eating servings from all the four food groups, but with smaller serving sizes, and elimination of excessive intake of processed sugars and their products. Eating regularly is important in order to maintain energy levels—the traditional three meals a day are best for most people. Including a daily multivitamin supplement is probably not necessary but is not harmful.

Fad diets for weight loss are common and usually ineffective. While many people initially lose weight, they gradually regain the weight when they become frustrated with the diet. This diet "yo-yo" effect is both physically and psychologically damaging for many people. Avoid diets that emphasize one kind of food—

they're not only boring but also dangerous to your health in the long run.

For those with severe, life-threatening obesity, rapid weight loss programs that involve modified fasting under a doctor's supervision are successful as long as:

- There is motivation to keep the weight off, and
- Emphasis is placed on modification of the person's eating habits (as soon as all the excess weight has been lost and food intake can be resumed) so that weight gain does not reoccur.

Do not go on fasts or modified fasts without a doctor's close supervision. Taking such a risk without proper supervision and evaluation can result in serious, life-threatening malnutrition and a variety of complications—including sudden death.

The tendency to obesity begins in infancy and childhood and is actually easier to prevent than to treat. Avoiding over-feeding infants and children and teaching healthy eating habits are essential. However, when this has failed and a person has become overweight, the best way to resolve the problem is through a sensible and reasonable approach: Follow a well-balanced reduction diet that provides enough energy to carry on usual activities and allows for about a two pound per week loss of weight (that's only a reduction of 7,000 calories per seven-day week from your usual caloric consumption); participate in an exercise program that helps with weight loss and also results in better physical fitness; and emphasize a change in eating habits designed to last for a lifetime.

Bibliography

General Nutrition

Brody, Jane. *Jane Brody's Nutrition Book*. New York: W. W. Norton, 1981.

Davidson, Stanley, Passmore, R., Brock, J. F., and Traswell, A. S. *Human Nutrition and Dietetics*. New York: Churchill Livingstone, 1979.

Food and Nutrition Board. *Recommended Dietary Allowances*. 9th ed. Washington, D.C.: National Research Council, National Academy of Sciences, 1980.

Goodhart, R. S., and Shils, M. E. *Modern Nutrition in Health and Disease*. 6th ed. Philadelphia: Lea and Febiger, 1980.

Jenkins, D. J. A., et al. "Treatment of Diabetics with Guar Gum." *The Lancet* 2 (1977):779 + .

McWilliams, Margaret. *Nutrition for the Growing Years*. New York: John Wiley & Sons, 1980.

Nutrition Search, Inc. *Nutrition Almanac*. New York: McGraw-Hill Book Company, 1979.

Pennington, Jean, and Church, Helen N. *Food Values of Portions Commonly Used*. 13th ed. Philadelphia: J. B. Lippincott Company, 1980.

Phillips, David A. *Guidebook to Nutritional Factors in Foods*. Santa Barbara, Calif.: Woodbridge Press Publishing Company, 1979.

Prince, Francine. *Diet for Life*. New York: Simon and Schuster, 1981.

Robinson, Corinne Hogden. *Normal and Therapeutic Nutrition*. New York: Macmillan Publishing Company, 1977.

Scarpa, I. S., Kiefer, Helen Chilton, Garmon, Gwenn, and Tatum, Rita, contributing eds. *Sourcebook on Food and Nutrition*. Chicago: Marquis Academic Media, 1980.

Suitor, Carol West. *Nutrition: Principles and Application in Health Promotion.* Philadelphia: J. B. Lippincott Company, 1980.

Toufexis, Anastasia. "Taming the No. 1 Killer." *Time* 117 (June 1, 1981):52 + .

U.S. Department of Agriculture. *Nutritive Value of Foods.* Washington, D.C.: U.S. Government Printing Office, April 1981.

U.S. Department of Health, Education and Welfare. *Using Nutrition Labels with Food Exchange Lists.* Pub. No. (FDA) 77:2072. Washington, D.C.: U.S. Government Printing Office.

U.S. Senate Select Committee on Nutrition and Human Needs. *Diet Related to Killer Diseases.* Washington, D.C.: U.S. Government Printing Office, January 1977.

——. *Diet Related to Killer Diseases, II, Part 1. Cardiovascular Disease.* February 1977.

——. *Diet Related to Killer Diseases, II, Part 2. Obesity.* February 1977.

——. *Dietary Goals for the United States—Supplemental Views.* Washington, D.C.: U.S. Government Printing Office, November 1977.

Winick, Myron. *Nutrition in Health and Disease.* New York: John Wiley & Sons, 1980.

Additives

Block, Zenas. *It's All on the Label: Understanding Food, Additives and Nutrition.* Boston: Little, Brown and Company, 1981.

Hopkins, Harold. "The Color Additive Scoreboard." *FDA Consumer* (March 1980):24–27.

Jacobson, Michael F. *Eater's Digest: The Consumer's Factbook of Food Additives.* New York: Doubleday & Co., 1976.

Maga, Joseph A. "Food Additive Toxicology." In *Survey of Contemporary Toxicology.* Vol. 1. Edited by Anthony T. Tu. New York: John Wiley & Sons, 1980.

Robbins, William. *The American Food Scandal.* New York: William Morrow & Company, 1974.

Fats

Flynn, Margaret A. "The Cholesterol Controversy." *Contemporary Nutrition* 3 (1978):1–2.

Gotto, Antonio M., Jr. "Is Atherosclerosis Reversible?" *Journal of the American Dietetic Association* 70 (1977):602.

Leverton, Ruth M. *Fats in the Diet.* Agricultural Information Bulletin 361. Washington, D.C.: U.S. Department of Agriculture, Superintendent of Documents, 1976.

Mattson, Fred H. "Fat." In *Nutrition Reviews' Present Knowledge in Nutrition.* 4th ed. Washington, D.C.: The Nutrition Foundation, 1976.

Wein, E. E., and Wilcox, E. B. "Serum Cholesterol from Pre-Adolescence Through Young Adulthood." *Journal of the American Dietetic Association* 61 (1972):155.

Fiber

Burkitt, Denis P. "The Link Between Low-Fiber Diets and Disease." *Human Nature* 1 (December 1978):34 + .

Galton, Lawrence. *The Truth About Fiber in Your Food.* New York: Crown Publishers, 1976.

Hegsted, D. M. "Food and Fiber: Evidence from Experimental Animals." *Nutrition Reviews* 35 (1977):45.

Van Soest, Peter. "The Secret My Friends Is the Fiber." *Human Ecology Forum* 6 (1976).

Van Soest, P. J., and Robertson, J. B. "What Is Fiber and Fiber in Food." *Nutrition Reviews* 35 (1977):12.

Fluids

Lecos, Chris. "Caution Light on Caffeine." *FDA Consumer* (October 1980):6 + .

Phillips, John H. "Chemical Pollutants in Water." In *Survey of Contemporary Toxicology.* Vol. 1. Edited by Anthony T. Tu. New York: John Wiley & Sons, 1980.

Safe Drinking Water Committee. *Drinking Water and Health.* Washington, D.C.: National Academy of Sciences, 1977.

Timson, John. "Is Coffee Safe to Drink?" *Human Nature* 1 (December 1978):56 + .

Protein

Broquist, H. P. "Amino Acid Metabolism." *Nutrition Reviews* 34 (1976):289–293.

Chopra, Joginder, Forbes, Allan L., and Habicht, Jean-Pierre. "Protein in the U.S. Diet." *Journal of the American Dietetic Association* 72 (March 1978):253 + .

Hegsted, D. M. "Protein Needs and Possible Modifications of the American Diet." *Journal of the American Dietetic Association* 68 (1976):317–320.

Olson, R. E., ed. *Protein-Caloric Malnutrition.* New York: Academic Press, 1975.

Palombo, John D., and Blackburn, G. L. "Human Protein Requirements." *Contemporary Nutrition* 5 (1980):1–2.

Wait, B. "Protein Intake of Well-Nourished Children and Adolescents." *American Journal of Clinical Nutrition* 26 (1973):1303.

Sodium

Dahl, L. K. "Salt and Hypertension." *American Journal of Clinical Nutrition* 25 (1972):231.

Meneely, G. R., and Battarbee, H. D. "Sodium and Potassium." *Nutrition Reviews* 34 (1976):225.

Morgan, T., et al. "Hypertension Treated by Salt Restriction." *The Lancet* 1 (1978):227.

Wallis, Claudia. "Salt: A New Villain?" *Time* 119 (March 15, 1982):64 + .

Sugar

Abrahamson, E. M., and Pezet, A. W. *Body, Mind & Sugar.* New York: Avon Books, 1977.

Behan, Kathy P. "Is Sugar Really Bad for You?" *Mademoiselle* (January 1982):65.

Burkitt, D. P., and Trowell, H. C. *Refined Carbohydrate Foods and Disease.* New York: Academic Press, 1975.

Danowski, T. S. "Sugar and Disease." *Contemporary Nutrition* 3 (December 1978).

———. *The Hypoglycemia Syndromes.* Pittsburgh: Harper Press, 1978.

Duffy, William. *Sugar Blues.* New York: Warner Books, 1975.

Lecos, Chris. "Food Labels and the Sugar Recognition Factor." *FDA Consumer* (April 1980):3–5.

———. "Fructose: Questionable Diet Aid." *FDA Consumer* (March 1980):21–23.

———. "Sugar: How Sweet It Is—And Isn't." *FDA Consumer* (February 1980):22–23.

Makinen, K. K., and Philosophy, L. "The Role of Sucrose and Other Sugars in the Development of Dental Caries." *Internal Dentistry Journal* 22 (1972):363.

"New Sugar, New Fat/New Thoughts." *Health* (March 1982):28+.

Ross, Shirley. *The Complete Carbohydrate Handbook.* New York: William Morrow & Company, 1981.

Yudkin, John. *Sweet and Dangerous.* New York: Bantam Books, 1972.

Vitamins & Minerals

Adams, Ruth. *The Complete Home Guide to All the Vitamins.* New York: Larchmont Books, 1972.

Appledorf, H., and Kelly, L. S. "Proximate and Mineral Content of Fast Foods." *Journal of the American Dietetic Association* 74 (1979):35.

Cook, James D. "Food Iron Availability." *Food and Nutrition News* 49 (February 1978):1, 4.

Ebon, Martin. *Which Vitamins Do You Need?* New York: Bantam Books, 1974.

Katz, Marcella. *Vitamins, Food, and Your Health.* Public Affairs Committee, 1975.

Mindell, Earl. *Vitamin Bible.* New York: Rawson, Wade Publishers, 1980.

Tuman, R. W., and Doisy, R. J. "The Role of Trace Elements in Human Nutrition and Metabolism." In *Sourcebook on Food and Nutrition.* 2nd ed. Edited by I. S. Scarpa and H. C. Kiefer. Chicago: Marquis Academic Media, 1980.

Underwood, Eric J. "Trace Element Imbalances of Interest to the Dietitian." *Journal of the American Dietetic Association* 72 (February 1978): 177-179.

Wong, N. P., La Croix, D. E., and Alford, John A. "Mineral Content of Dairy Products." *Journal of the American Dietetic Association* 72 (June 1978):608-611.

Appendix

Appendix I

NUTRITIVE VALUES OF THE EDIBLE PART OF FOODS

(A dot ● denotes lack of reliable data for a constituent
believed to be present in measurable amount;
the letter T indicates that a trace of the constituent in question is present.)

Nutrients in Indicated Quantity

Foods, approximate measures, units and weight (edible part unless footnotes indicate otherwise)	Water	Food Energy	Protein	Fat (Total)	Saturated (Total)	Unsaturated Oleic	Linoleic	Carbohydrate
	Grams	Percent	Calories	Grams	Grams	Grams	Grams	Grams	Grams
Almonds, shelled:								
Chopped (about 130 almonds), 1 cup	130	5	775	24	70	5.6	47.7	12.8	25
Apples, raw, unpeeled, 3¼ in. diam. (about 2 per lb. with cores), 1 apple	212	84	125	T	1	●	●	●	31

Foods, approximate measures, units and weight (edible part unless footnotes indicate otherwise)	Water Percent	Food Energy Calories	Protein Grams	Fat (Total) Grams	Saturated (Total) Grams	Unsaturated Oleic Grams	Linoleic Grams	Carbohydrate Grams
Grams	*Percent*	*Calories*	*Grams*	*Grams*	*Grams*	*Grams*	*Grams*	*Grams*
Apricots:								
Raw, without pits (about 12 per lb. with pits), 3 apricots 107	85	55	1	T	•	•	•	14
Asparagus, green:								
Cooked, drained:								
Spears, ½-in. diam. at base:								
From raw, 4 spears 60	94	10	1	T	•	•	•	2
Bacon, (20 slices per lb. raw), broiled or fried, crisp, 2 slices 15	8	85	4	8	2.5	3.7	.7	T
Bagel, Egg, 3-in. diam., 1 bagel 55	32	165	6	2	.5	.9	.8	28
Banana without peel (about 2½ per lb. with peel), 1 banana 119	76	100	1	T	•	•	•	26
Beans:								
Baby Limas, 1 cup 180	69	210	13	T	•	•	•	40
Snap:								
Green:								
From raw (cuts and French style), 1 cup 125	92	30	2	T	•	•	•	7

Yellow or wax:									
From raw (cuts and French, style), 1 cup	125	93	30	2	T	•	•	•	6
Bean sprouts (mung):									
Raw, 1 cup	105	89	35	4	T	•	•	•	7
Beef, cooked:									
Cuts braised, simmered or pot roasted:									
Lean and fat (piece, 2½ by 2½ by ¾ in.), 3 oz.	85	53	245	23	16	6.8	6.5	.4	0
Ground Beef, broiled:									
Lean with 10% fat, 3 oz. or patty 3 by ⅝ in.	85	60	185	23	10	4.0	3.9	.3	0
Roast, oven cooked, no liquid added:									
Relatively fat, such as rib:									
Lean and fat (2 pieces, 4⅛ by 2¼ by ¼ in., 3 oz.	85	40	375	17	33	14.0	13.6	.8	0
Roast, oven cooked, no liquid added:									
Relatively lean, such as heel of round:									
Lean and fat (2 pieces, 4⅛ by 2¼ by ¼ in.), 3 oz.	85	62	165	25	7	2.8	2.7	.2	0

Foods, approximate measures, units and weight (edible part unless footnotes indicate otherwise)		Water	Food Energy	Protein	Fat (Total)	Saturated (Total)	Unsaturated Oleic	Linoleic	Carbohydrate
	Grams	Percent	Calories	Grams	Grams	Grams	Grams	Grams	Grams
Steak:									
Relatively fat, sirloin, broiled:									
Lean and fat (piece, 2½ by ¾ in.), 3 oz.	85	44	330	20	27	11.3	11.1	.6	0
Relatively lean, round, braised:									
Lean and fat (piece, 4⅛ by 2¼ by ½ in.), 3 oz.	85	55	220	24	13	5.5	5.2	.4	0
Beer, 12 fl. oz.	360	92	150	1	0	0	0	0	14
Beets:									
Whole beets, 2-in. diam., 2 beets	100	91	30	1	T	•	•	•	7
Biscuits, baking powder, 2-in. diam. (enriched flour, vegetable shortening):									
From mix, 1 biscuit	28	29	90	2	3	.6	1.1	.7	15
Blackeyed peas, dry, cooked (with residual cooking liquid), 1 cup	250	80	190	13	1	•	•	•	35

Food	Grams	Water (%)	Food energy	Protein (g)	Fat (g)			Carbohydrate
Blackberries, raw, 1 cup	144	85	85	2	1	•	•	•	19
Blueberries, raw, 1 cup	145	83	90	1	1	•	•	•	22
Bluefish, baked with butter or margarine, 3 oz.	85	68	135	22	4	•	•	•	0
Bologna, slice (8 per 8-oz. pkg.), 1 slice	28	56	85	3	8	3.0	3.4	.5	T
Braunschweiger, slice (6 per 6-oz. pkg.), 1 slice	28	53	90	4	8	2.6	3.4	.8	1
Brazil nuts, shelled (6-8 large kernels), 1 oz.	28	5	185	4	19	4.8	6.2	7.1	3
Breads								
Cracked-wheat bread (¾ enriched wheat flour, ¼ cracked wheat): Slice (18 per loaf), 1 slice	25	35	65	2	1	.1	.2	.2	13
French or Vienna bread, enriched: Slice: French (5 by 2½ by 1 in.), 1 slice	35	31	100	3	1	.2	.4	.4	19
Vienna (4¾ by 4 by ½ in.), 1 slice	25	31	75	2	1	.2	.3	.3	14
Italian bread, enriched: Slice, 4½ by 3¼ by ¾ in., 1 slice	30	32	85	3	T	T	T	.1	17

Foods, approximate measures, units and weight (edible part unless footnotes indicate otherwise)		Water	Food Energy	Protein	Fat (Total)	Saturated (Total)	Unsaturated Oleic	Linoleic	Carbohydrate
	Grams	Percent	Calories	Grams	Grams	Grams	Grams	Grams	Grams
Raisin bread, enriched:									
Slice (18 per loaf), 1 slice	25	35	65	2	1	.2	.3	.2	13
Rye Bread:									
American, light (⅔ enriched wheat flour, ⅓ rye flour):									
Slice (4¾ by 3¾ by 7/16 in.), 1 slice	25	36	60	2	T	T	T	.1	13
Pumpernickel (⅔ rye flour, ⅓ enriched wheat flour):									
Slice (5 by 4 by ⅜ in.), 1 slice	32	34	80	3	T	.1	T	.2	17
White Bread, enriched:									
Soft-crumb type:									
Slice (18 per loaf), 1 slice	25	36	70	2	1	.2	.3	.3	13
Slice, toasted, 1 slice	22	25	70	2	1	.2	.3	.3	13
Firm-crumb type:									
Slice (20 per loaf), 1 slice	23	35	65	2	1	.2	.3	.3	12
Slice, toasted, 1 slice	20	24	65	2	1	.2	.3	.3	12

Whole-wheat bread:									
Soft-crumb type:									
Slice (16 per loaf), 1 slice	28	36	65	3	1	.1	.2	.2	14
Slice, toasted, 1 slice	24	24	65	3	1	.1	.2	.2	14
Firm-crumb type:									
Slice (18 per loaf), 1 slice	25	36	60	3	1	.1	.2	.3	12
Slice, toasted, 1 slice	21	24	60	3	1	.1	.2	.3	12
Breakfast cereals:									
Hot type, cooked:									
Farina, quick-cooking, enriched, 1 cup	245	89	105	3	T	T	T	.1	22
Oatmeal or rolled oats, 1 cup	240	87	130	5	2	.4	.8	.9	23
Wheat, whole-meal, 1 cup	245	88	110	4	1	•	•	•	23
Ready-to-eat:									
Bran flakes (40% bran), added sugar, salt, iron, vitamins, 1 cup	35	3	105	4	1	•	•	•	28
Corn flakes:									
Plain, added sugar, salt, iron, vitamins, 1 cup	25	4	95	2	T	•	•	•	21
Sugar-coated, added salt, iron, vitamins, 1 cup	40	2	155	2	T	•	•	•	37

Foods, approximate measures, units and weight (edible part unless footnotes indicate otherwise)		Water Percent	Food Energy Calories	Protein Grams	Fat (Total) Grams	Saturated (Total) Grams	Unsaturated Oleic Grams	Linoleic Grams	Carbohydrate Grams
	Grams								
Corn, puffed, plain, added sugar, salt, iron, vitamins, 1 cup	20	4	80	2	1	•	•	•	16
Corn, shredded, added sugar, salt, iron, thiamin, niacin, 1 cup	25	3	95	2	T	•	•	•	22
Oats, puffed, added sugar, salt, minerals, vitamins, 1 cup	25	3	100	3	1	•	•	•	19
Rice, puffed: Plain, added iron, thiamin, niacin, 1 cup	15	4	60	1	T	•	•	•	13
Wheat flakes, added sugar, salt, iron, vitamins, 1 cup	30	4	105	3	T	•	•	•	24
Wheat, puffed: Plain, added iron, thiamin, niacin, 1 cup	15	3	55	2	T	•	•	•	12
Presweetened, added salt, iron, vitamins, 1 cup	38	3	140	3	T	•	•	•	33

Food, approximate measure									
Wheat, shredded, plain, 1 oblong biscuit or ½ cup spoon-size biscuits	25	7	90	2	1	•	•	•	20
Wheat germ without salt and sugar, toasted, 1 tbsp.	6	4	25	2	1	•	•	•	3
Broccoli:									
From stalk, medium size, 1 stalk	180	91	45	6	1	•	•	•	8
Brussels sprouts, cooked, drained:									
From raw, 7-8 sprouts (1¼ to 1½ in. diam.), 1 cup	155	88	55	7	1	•	•	•	10
Butter:									
Tablespoon (about ⅛ stick), 1 tbsp.	14	16	100	T	12	7.2	2.9	.3	T
Whipped (6 sticks or two 8-oz. containers per lb.): Tablespoon (about ⅛ stick), 1 tbsp.	9	16	65	T	8	4.7	1.9	.2	T
Cabbage:									
Raw, coarsely shredded or sliced, 1 cup	70	92	15	1	T	•	•	•	4
Cooked, drained, 1 cup	145	94	30	2	T	•	•	•	6
Red, raw, coarsely shredded or sliced, 1 cup	70	90	20	1	T	•	•	•	5

Foods, approximate measures, units and weight (edible part unless footnotes indicate otherwise)		Water	Food Energy	Protein	Fat (Total)	Saturated (Total)	Unsaturated Oleic	Linoleic	Carbohydrate
	Grams	Percent	Calories	Grams	Grams	Grams	Grams	Grams	Grams
Savory, raw, coarsely shredded or sliced, 1 cup	70	92	15	2	T	•	•	•	3
Cakes made from cake mixes with enriched flour:									
Angelfood:									
Whole cake (9¾ in. diam. tube cake), 1 cake	635	34	1,645	36	1	•	•	•	377
Coffeecake:									
Whole cake (7¾ by 5⅝ by 1¼ in.), 1 cake	430	30	1,385	27	41	11.7	16.3	8.8	225
Cupcakes, made with egg, milk, 2½ in. diam.:									
Without icing, 1 cupcake	25	26	90	1	3	.8	1.2	.7	14
With chocolate icing, 1 cupcake	36	22	130	2	5	2.0	.16	.6	21
Devil's food with chocolate icing:									
Whole, 2 layer cake (8 or 9 in. diam.), 1 cake	1,107	24	3,755	49	136	50.0	44.9	17.0	645

Food								
Cupcake, 2½ in. diam, 1 cupcake	35	24	120	2	4	1.6	.14	.5	20
Gingerbread: Whole cake (8 in. square), 1 cake	570	37	1,575	18	39	9.7	16.6	10.0	291
White, 2 layer with chocolate icing: Whole cake (8 or 9 in. diam.), 1 cake	1,140	21	4,000	44	122	48.2	16.4	20.0	716
Yellow, 2 layer with chocolate icing: Whole cake (8 or 9 in. diam.), 1 cake	1,108	26	3,735	45	125	47.8	47.8	10.3	638
Cantaloupe, orange-fleshed (with rind and seed cavity, 5 in. diam., 2⅓ lb.), ½ melon with rind	477	91	80	2	T	•	•	•	20
Carrots: Raw, without crowns and tips, scraped: Whole, 7½ by 1⅛ in. or strips, 2½ to 3 in. long, 1 carrot or 18 strips	72	88	30	1	T	•	•	•	7

Foods, approximate measures, units and weight (edible part unless footnotes indicate otherwise)	Grams	Water Percent	Food Energy Calories	Protein Grams	Fat (Total) Grams	Saturated (Total) Grams	Unsaturated Oleic Grams	Unsaturated Linoleic Grams	Carbohydrate Grams
Cooked (crosswise cuts), drained, 1 cup	155	91	50	1	T	•	•	•	11
Cashew nuts, roasted in oil, 1 cup	140	5	785	24	64	12.9	36.8	10.2	41
Cauliflower:									
Cooked, from raw (flower buds), 1 cup	125	93	30	3	T	•	•	•	5
Celery, Pascal type, raw:									
Stalk, large outer, 8 by 1½ in. at root end, 1 stalk	40	94	5	T	T	•	•	•	2
Cheese:									
Natural:									
Blue, 1 oz.	28	42	100	6	8	5.3	1.9	.2	1
Camembert (3 wedges per 4 oz. container), 1 wedge	38	52	115	8	9	5.8	2.2	.2	T
Cheddar:									
Cut pieces, 1 oz.	28	37	115	7	9	6.1	2.1	.2	T
Cottage (curd not pressed down):									

Creamed (cottage cheese, 4% fat):								
Large curd, 1 cup	225	79	235	28	10	6.4	2.4	.2	6
Small curd, 1 cup	210	79	220	26	9	6.0	2.2	.2	6
Low fat (1%), 1 cup	226	82	165	28	2	1.5	.5	.1	6
Cream, 1 oz.	28	54	100	2	10	6.2	2.4	.2	1
Mozzarella, made with:								
Whole milk, 1 oz.	28	48	90	6	7	4.4	4.7	.2	1
Part skim milk, 1 oz.	28	49	80	8	5	3.1	1.2	.1	1
Parmesan, grated:								
Tablespoon, 1 tbsp.	5	18	25	2	2	1.0	.4	T	T
Provolone, 1 oz.	28	41	100	7	8	4.8	4.7	.1	1
Ricotta, made with:								
Whole milk, 1 cup	246	72	428	28	32	20.4	7.1	.7	7
Part skim milk, 1 cup	246	74	340	28	19	12.1	4.7	.5	13
Romano, 1 oz.	28	31	110	9	8	•	•	•	1
Swiss, 1 oz.	28	37	105	8	8	5.0	1.7	.2	1
Pasteurized process cheese:								
American, 1 oz.	28	39	105	6	9	5.6	2.1	.2	T
Swiss, 1 oz.	28	42	95	7	7	4.5	1.7	.1	1
Cherries:								
Sweet, raw, without pits and stems, 10 cherries	68	80	45	1	T	•	•	•	12

Foods, approximate measures, units and weight (edible part unless footnotes indicate otherwise)		Water	Food Energy	Protein	Fat (Total)	Saturated (Total)	Unsaturated Oleic	Linoleic	Carbohydrate
	Grams	Percent	Calories	Grams	Grams	Grams	Grams	Grams	Grams
Chicken, cooked:									
Breast, fried, bones removed, ½ breast (3⅓ oz. with bones), 2¾ oz.	79	58	160	26	5	1.4	1.8	1.1	1
Drumstick, fried, bones removed (2 oz. with bones), 13 oz.	38	55	90	12	4	1.1	1.3	.9	T
Half broiler, broiled, bones removed (10½ oz. with bones), 6¼ oz.	176	71	240	42	7	2.2	2.5	1.3	0
Chili con carne with beans, canned, 1 cup	255	72	340	19	16	7.5	6.8	.3	31
Chocolate:									
Bitter or baking, 1 oz.	28	2	145	3	15	8.9	4.9	.4	8
Semisweet, see Candy, chocolate.									
Chocolate milk (commercial): Regular, 1 cup	250	82	210	8	8	5.3	2.2	.2	26

Food	g	%	cal	g	g	g	g	g	g
Lowfat (1%), 1 cup	250	85	160	8	3	1.5	.7	.1	26
Clams: Raw, meat only, 3 oz.	85	82	65	11	1	•	•	•	2
Coconut meat, fresh: Shredded or grated, not pressed down, 1 cup	80	51	275	3	28	24.8	1.6	.5	8
Cola drink, 12 fl. oz.	369	90	145	0	0	0	0	0	37
Cookies made with enriched flour:									
Brownies with nuts: Home-prepared, 1¾ by 1¾ by ⅞ in.: From home recipe, 1 brownie	20	10	95	1	6	1.5	3.0	1.2	10
From commercial recipe, 1 brownie	20	11	85	1	4	.9	1.4	1.3	13
Chocolate Chip: Commercial, 2¼ in. diam., ⅜ in. thick, 4 cookies	42	3	200	2	9	2.8	2.9	2.2	29
From home recipe, 2⅓ in. diam., 4 cookies	40	3	205	2	12	3.5	4.5	2.9	24
Gingersnaps, 2 in. diam., ¼ in. thick, 4 cookies	28	3	90	2	2	.7	1.0	.6	22
Macaroons, 2¾ in. diam., ¼ in. thick, 2 cookies	38	4	180	2	9	•	•	•	25

Foods, approximate measures, units and weight (edible part unless footnotes indicate otherwise)		Water	Food Energy	Protein	Fat (Total)	Saturated (Total)	Unsaturated Oleic	Linoleic	Carbohydrate
	Grams	Percent	Calories	Grams	Grams	Grams	Grams	Grams	Grams
Oatmeal with raisins, 2⅝ in. diam., ¼ in. thick, 4 cookies	52	3	235	3	8	2.0	3.3	2.0	38
Sandwich type (chocolate or vanilla), 1¾ in. diam., ⅜ in. thick, 4 cookies	40	2	200	2	9	2.2	3.9	2.2	28
Vanilla Wafers, 1¾ in. diam., ¼ in. thick, 10 cookies	40	3	185	2	6	•	•	•	30
Corn, sweet: Cooked, drained: From raw, ear 5 by 1¾ in., 1 ear	140	74	70	2	1	•	•	•	16
Crabmeat (white or king), canned, not pressed down, 1 cup	135	77	135	24	3	.6	.4	.1	12
Crackers: Graham, plain, 2½ in. square, 2 crackers	14	6	55	1	1	.3	.5	.3	10

Food	Grams	Water %	Calories						
Rye wafers, whole-grain, 1⅞ by 3½ in., 2 wafers	13	6	45	2	T	•	•	•	10
Saltines, made with enriched flour, 4 crackers or 1 packet	11	4	50	1	1	.3	.5	.4	8
Cranberry juice cocktail, bottled, sweetened, 1 cup	253	83	165	T	T	•	•	•	42
Cranberry sauce, sweetened, canned, strained, 1 cup	277	62	405	T	1	•	•	•	104
Cream products, imitation (made with vegetable fat): Sweet: Creamers:									
Liquid (frozen), 1 cup	245	77	335	2	24	22.8	.3	T	28
Powdered, 1 cup	94	2	515	5	33	30.6	.9	T	52
Whipped topping:									
Frozen, 1 cup	75	50	240	1	19	16.3	1.0	.2	17
Pressurized, 1 cup	70	60	185	1	16	13.2	1.4	.2	11
Cream, sour, 1 cup	230	71	495	7	48	30.0	12.1	1.1	10
Cream, sweet: Half-and-Half (cream and milk), 1 cup	242	81	315	7	28	17.3	7.0	.6	10
Light, coffee, or table, 1 cup	240	74	470	6	46	28.8	11.7	1.0	9

Foods, approximate measures, units and weight (edible part unless footnotes indicate otherwise)		Water	Food Energy	Protein	Fat (Total)	Saturated (Total)	Unsaturated Oleic	Linoleic	Carbohydrate
	Grams	Percent	Calories	Grams	Grams	Grams	Grams	Grams	Grams
Whipping, unwhipped (volume about double when whipped):									
Light, 1 cup	239	64	700	5	74	46.2	18.3	1.5	7
Heavy, 1 cup	238	58	820	5	88	54.8	22.2	2.0	7
Whipped topping, (pressurized), 1 cup	60	61	155	2	13	8.3	3.4	.3	7
Cucumber slices, ⅛ in. thick (large, 2⅛ in. diam.; small, 1¾ in. diam.):									
With peel, 6 large or 8 small slices	28	95	5	T	T	•	•	•	1
Custard, baked, 1 cup	265	77	305	14	15	6.8	5.4	.7	29
Dates:									
Whole, without pits, 10 dates	80	23	220	2	T	•	•	•	58
Doughnuts, made with enriched flour:									
Cake type, plain, 2½ in. diam., 1 in. high, 1 doughnut	25	24	100	1	5	1.2	2.0	1.1	13

Food									
Eggnog (commercial), 1 cup	254	74	340	10	19	11.3	5.0	.6	34
Eggs, large (24 oz. per dozen): Cooked:									
Fried in butter, 1 egg	46	72	85	5	6	2.4	2.2	.6	1
Hard-cooked, shell removed, 1 egg	50	75	80	6	6	1.7	2.0	.6	1
Poached, 1 egg	50	74	80	6	6	1.7	2.0	.6	1
Scrambled (milk added) in butter. Also omelet, 1 egg	64	76	95	6	7	2.8	2.3	.6	1
Endive, curly (including escarole), raw, small pieces, 1 cup	50	93	10	1	T	•	•	•	2
Fats, cooking (vegetable shortenings), 1 cup	200	0	1,770	0	200	48.8	88.2	48.4	0
1 tbsp.	13	0	110	0	13	3.2	5.7	3.1	0
Filberts (hazelnuts), chopped (about 80 kernels), 1 cup	115	6	730	14	72	5.1	55.2	7.3	19
Fish sticks, breaded, cooked, frozen (stick, 4 by 1 by ½ in.), 1 fish stick or 1 oz.	28	66	50	5	3	•	•	•	2
Frankfurter (8 per 1 lb. pkg.), cooked (reheated), 1 frankfurter	56	57	170	7	15	5.6	6.5	1.2	1
Fruit cocktail, canned, in heavy syrup, 1 cup	255	80	195	1	T	•	•	•	50

233

Foods, approximate measures, units and weight (edible part unless footnotes indicate otherwise)		Water	Food Energy	Protein	Fat (Total)	Saturated (Total)	Unsaturated Oleic	Linoleic	Carbohydrate
	Grams	Percent	Calories	Grams	Grams	Grams	Grams	Grams	Grams
Fruit-flavored sodas and Tom Collins mixer, 12 fl. oz.	372	88	170	0	0	0	0	0	45
Gelatin dessert prepared with gelatin dessert powder and water, 1 cup	240	84	140	4	0	0	0	0	34
Ginger ale, 12 fl. oz.	366	92	115	0	0	0	0	0	29
Grape drink, canned, 1 cup	250	86	135	T	T	•	•	•	35
Grapefruit juice:									
Canned, white:									
Unsweetened, 1 cup	247	89	100	1	T	•	•	•	24
Frozen, concentrate, unsweetened:									
Diluted with 3 parts water by volume, 1 cup	247	89	100	1	T	•	•	•	24
Grapefruit:									
Raw, medium, 3¾ in. diam. (about 1 lb. 1 oz.):									
White, ½ grapefruit with peel	241	89	45	1	T	•	•	•	12

Food	Weight (g)	Water (%)	Food energy (cal)	Protein (g)	Fat (g)	Saturated	Oleic	Linoleic	Carbohydrate (g)
Grape juice:									
Canned or bottled, 1 cup	253	83	165	1	T	•	•		42
Frozen concentrate, sweetened: Diluted with 3 parts water by volume, 1 cup	250	86	135	1	T	•	•		33
Grapes; European type (adherent skin) raw:									
Thompson Seedless, 10 grapes	50	81	35	T	T	•	•		9
Tokay and Emperor seeded types, 10 grapes	60	81	40	T	T	•	•		10
Haddock, breaded, fried, 3 oz.	85	66	140	17	5	1.4	2.2	1.2	5
Heart, beef, lean, braised, 3 oz.	85	61	160	27	5	1.5	1.1	.6	1
Honey, strained or extracted, 1 tbsp.	21	17	65	T	0	0	0	0	17
Honeydew (with rind and seed cavity, 6½ in. diam., 5¼ lb.), 1/10 melon with rind	226	91	50	1	T	•	•		11
Ice Cream:									
Regular (about 11% fat):									
Hardened, 1 cup	133	61	270	5	14	8.9	3.6	.3	32
Soft serve (frozen custard), 1 cup	173	60	375	7	23	13.5	5.9	.6	38
Rich (about 16% fat), hardened, 1 cup	148	59	350	4	24	14.7	6.0	.5	32

Foods, approximate measures, units and weigh (edible part unless footnotes indicate otherwise)		Water Percent	Food Energy Calories	Protein Grams	Fat (Total) Grams	Saturated (Total) Grams	Unsaturated Oleic Grams	Linoleic Grams	Carbohydrate Grams
	Grams								
Ice Milk:									
Hardened (about 4.3% fat), 1 cup	131	69	185	5	6	3.5	1.4	.1	29
Soft serve (about 2.6% fat), 1 cup	175	70	225	8	5	2.9	1.2	.1	38
Jams and preserves, 1 tbsp.	20	29	55	T	T	•	•	•	14
Jellies, 1 tbsp.	18	29	50	T	T	•	•	•	13
Kale, cooked, drained:									
From raw (leaves without stems and midribs), 1 cup	110	88	45	5	1	•	•	•	7
Lamb, cooked:									
Chop, rib (cut 3 per lb. with bone), broiled:									
Lean and fat, 3.1 oz.	89	43	360	18	32	14.8	12.1	1.2	0
Leg, roasted:									
Lean and fat (2 pieces, 4⅛ by 2¼ by ¼ in.), 3 oz.	85	54	235	22	16	7.3	6.0	.6	0

	Grams	Water (%)							
Shoulder, roasted:									
Lean and fat (3 pieces), 2½ by 2½ by ¼ in.), 3 oz.	85	50	285	18	23	10.8	8.8	.9	0
Lard, 1 tbsp.	13	0	115	0	13	5.1	5.3	1.3	0
Lemonade concentrate, frozen:									
Diluted with 4⅓ parts water by volume, 1 cup	248	89	105	T	T	•	•	•	28
Lemon juice:									
Raw, 1 cup	244	91	60	1	T	•	•	•	20
Lemon, raw, size 165, without peel and seeds (about 4 per lb. with peels and seeds), 1 lemon	74	90	20	1	T	•	•	•	6
Lentils, whole, cooked, 1 cup	200	72	210	16	T	•	•	•	39
Lettuce, raw:									
Butterhead, as Boston types: Leaves, 1 outer or 2 inner or 3 heart leaves	14	95	T	T	T	•	•	•	T
Crisphead, as Iceberg: Pieces, chopped or shredded, 1 cup	55	96	5	T	T	•	•	•	2
Looseleaf (bunching varieties including romain or cos), chopped or shredded pieces, 1 cup	55	94	10	1	T	•	•	•	2

Foods, approximate measures, units and weight (edible part unless footnotes indicate otherwise)		Water	Food Energy	Protein	Fat (Total)	Fat (Total) Saturated (Total)	Unsaturated Oleic	Unsaturated Linoleic	Carbohydrate
	Grams	Percent	Calories	Grams	Grams	Grams	Grams	Grams	Grams
Limeade concentrate, frozen:									
Diluted with 4⅓ parts water by volume, 1 cup	247	89	100	T	T	•	•	•	27
Lime juice:									
Raw, 1 cup	246	90	65	1	T	•	•	•	22
Liquor, gin, rum, vodka, whisky:									
80 proof, 1½ fl. oz. jigger	42	67	95	•	•	0	0	0	T
86 proof, 1½ fl. oz. jigger	42	64	105	•	•	0	0	0	T
90 proof, 1½ fl. oz. jigger	42	62	110	•	•	0	0	0	T
Liver, beef, fried (slice, 6½ by 2⅜ by ⅜ in.), 3 oz.	85	56	195	22	9	2.5	3.5	.9	5
Macaroni, enriched, cooked (cut lengths, elbows, shells):									
Firm stage (hot), 1 cup	130	64	190	7	1	•	•	•	39
Tender stage:									
Cold macaroni, 1 cup	105	73	115	4	T	•	•	•	24
Hot macaroni, 1 cup	140	73	155	5	1	•	•	•	32

Margarine:									
Regular (1 brick or 4 sticks per lb.):									
Tablespoon (about ⅛ stick), 1 tbsp.	14	16	100	T	12	2.1	5.3	3.1	T
Whipped (6 sticks per lb.):									
Tablespoon (about ⅛ stick), 1 tbsp.	9	16	70	T	8	1.4	3.6	2.1	T
Meat, potted (beef, chicken, turkey), canned, 1 tbsp.	13	61	30	2	2	•	•	•	0
Milk:									
Fluid:									
Whole (3.3% fat), 1 cup	244	88	150	8	8	5.1	2.1	.2	11
Lowfat (2%):									
No milk solids added, 1 cup	244	89	120	8	5	2.9	1.2	.1	12
Lowfat (1%):									
No milk solids added, 1 cup	244	90	100	8	3	1.6	.7	.1	12
Nonfat (skim):									
No milk solids added, 1 cup	245	91	85	8	T	.3	.1	T	12
Buttermilk, 1 cup	245	90	100	8	2	1.3	.5	T	12
Canned:									
Evaporated, unsweetened:									
Whole milk, 1 cup	252	74	340	17	19	11.6	5.3	.4	25
Skim milk, 1 cup	255	79	200	19	1	.3	.1	T	29

239

Foods, approximate measures, units and weight (edible part unless footnotes indicate otherwise)		Water	Food Energy	Protein	Fat (Total)	Saturated (Total)	Unsaturated Oleic	Unsaturated Linoleic	Carbohydrate
	Grams	Percent	Calories	Grams	Grams	Grams	Grams	Grams	Grams
Sweetened, condensed, 1 cup	306	27	980	24	27	16.8	6.7	.7	166
Dried:									
Buttermilk, 1 cup	120	3	465	41	7	4.3	1.7	.2	59
Nonfat, instant:									
Cup, 1 cup	68	4	245	24	T	.3	.1	T	35
Muffins made with enriched flour:									
From home receipe:									
Blueberry, 2⅜ in. diam., 1½ in. high, 1 muffin	40	39	110	3	4	1.1	1.4	.7	17
Bran, 1 muffin	40	35	105	3	4	1.2	1.4	.8	17
Corn (enriched degermed cornmeal and flour), 2⅜ in. diam., 1½ in. high, 1 muffin	40	33	125	3	4	1.2	1.6	.9	19
Plain, 3 in. diam., 1½ in. high, 1 muffin	40	38	120	3	4	1.0	1.7	1.0	17

Mushrooms, raw sliced or chopped, 1 cup	70	90	20	2	•	•	•	•	3
Mustard, prepared yellow, 1 tsp. or individual serving pouch or cup	5	80	5	T	T	•	•	•	T
Mustard greens, without stems and midribs, cooked, drained, 1 cup	140	93	30	3	1	•	•	•	6
Noodles (egg), enriched, cooked, 1 cup	160	71	200	7	2	•	•	•	37
Oils, salad or cooking:								
Corn, 1 tbsp.	14	0	120	0	14	1.7	3.3	7.8	0
Olive, 1 tbsp.	14	0	120	0	14	1.9	9.7	1.1	0
Peanut, 1 tbsp.	14	0	120	0	14	2.3	6.2	4.2	0
Safflower, 1 tbsp.	14	0	120	0	14	1.3	1.6	10.0	0
Soybean oil, hydrogenated (partially hardened), 1 tbsp.	14	0	120	0	14	2.0	5.8	4.7	0
Soybean-cottonseed oil blend, hydrogenated, 1 cup	218	0	1,925	0	218	38.2	63.0	99.6	0
1 tbsp	14	0	120	0	14	2.4	3.9	6.2	0
Olives, pickled, canned:								
Green, 4 medium or 3 extra large or 2 giant	16	78	15	T	2	.2	1.2	.1	T
Ripe, Mission, 3 small or 2 large	10	73	15	T	2	.2	1.2	.1	T

Foods, approximate measures, units and weight (edible part unless footnotes indicate otherwise)		Water	Food Energy	Protein	Fat (Total)	Saturated (Total)	Unsaturated Oleic	Linoleic	Carbohydrate
	Grams	Percent	Calories	Grams	Grams	Grams	Grams	Grams	Grams
Onions:									
Mature:									
Raw:									
Chopped, 1 cup	170	89	65	3	T	●	●		15
Sliced, 1 cup	115	89	45	2	T	●	●	●	10
Cooked (whole or sliced), drained, 1 cup	210	92	60	3	T	●	●	●	14
Young green, bulb (⅜ in. diam.) and white portion of top, 6 onions	30	88	15	T	T	●	●	●	3
Orange and grapefruit juice:									
Frozen concentrate:									
Diluted with 3 parts water by volume, 1 cup	248	88	110	1	T	●	●	●	26
Orange juice:									
Raw, all varieties, 1 cup	248	88	110	2	T	●	●	●	26
Canned, unsweetened, 1 cup	249	87	120	2	T	●	●	●	28

Food	Grams	Water %	Food energy	Protein	Fat				
Frozen concentrate:									
Diluted with 3 parts water by volume, 1 cup	249	87	120	2	T	•	•	•	29
Oranges, all commercial varieties, raw:									
Whole, 2⅝ in. diam., without peel and seeds (about 2½ per lb. with peel and seeds), 1 orange	131	86	65	1	T	•	•	•	16
Sections without membranes, 1 cup	180	86	90	2	T	•	•	•	22
Oysters, raw, meat only (13-19 medium Selects), 1 cup	240	85	160	20	4	1.3	.2	.1	8
Pancakes, (4 in. diam.):									
Buckwheat, made from mix (with buckwheat and enriched flours) egg and milk added, 1 cake	27	58	55	2	2	.8	.9	.4	6
Plain:									
Made from mix with enriched flour, egg and milk added, 1 cake	27	51	60	2	2	.7	.7	.3	9
Parsley, raw, chopped, 1 tbsp.	4	85	T	T	T	•	•	•	T

243

244

Foods, approximate measures, units and weight (edible part unless footnotes indicate otherwise)		Water Percent	Food Energy Calories	Protein Grams	Fat (Total) Grams	Saturated (Total) Grams	Unsaturated Oleic Grams	Linoleic Grams	Carbohydrate Grams
	Grams								
Parsnips, cooked (diced or 2 in. lengths), 1 cup	155	82	100	2	1	•	•	•	23
Peaches:									
Raw:									
Whole, 2½ in. diam., peeled, pitted (about 4 per lb. with peels and pits), 1 peach	100	89	40	1	T				10
Sliced, 1 cup	170	89	65	1	T				16
Peanuts, roasted in oil, salted (whole, halves, chopped), 1 cup	144	2	840	37	72	13.7	33.0	20.7	27
Peanut butter, 1 tbsp.	16	2	95	4	8	1.5	3.7	2.3	3
Pears:									
Raw, with skin, cored: Bartlett, 2½ in. diam. (about 2½ per lb. with cores and stems), 1 pear	164	83	100	1	1	•	•	•	25

Food	Weight (g)	Water (%)	Food energy (cal.)	Protein (g)	Fat (g)				Carbohydrate (g)
Bosc, 2½ in. diam. (about 3 per lb. with cores and stems), 1 pear	141	83	85	1	1	•	•	•	22
D'Anjou, 3 in. diam. (about 2 per lb. with cores and stems), 1 pear	200	83	120	1	1	•	•	•	31
Peas, green:									
Frozen, cooked, drained, 1 cup	160	82	110	8	T	•	•	•	19
Peas, split, dry, cooked, 1 cup	200	70	230	16	1	•	•	•	42
Pecans, chopped or pieces (about 120 large halves), 1 cup	118	3	810	11	84	7.2	50.5	20.0	17
Peppers, hot, red, without seeds, dried (Ground chili powder, added seasonings), 1 tsp.	2	9	5	T	T	•	•	•	1
Peppers, sweet (about 5 per lb. whole), stems and seeds removed:									
Raw, 1 pod	74	93	15	1	T	•	•	•	4
Cooked, boiled, drained, 1 pod	73	95	15	1	T	•	•	•	3
Pickles, cucumber:									
Dill, medium, whole, 3¾ in. long, 1¼ in. diam., 1 pickle	65	93	5	T	T	•	•	•	1

Foods, approximate measures, units and weight (edible part unless footnotes indicate otherwise)		Water Percent	Food Energy Calories	Protein Grams	Fat (Total) Grams	Saturated (Total) Grams	Unsaturated Oleic Grams	Unsaturated Linoleic Grams	Carbohydrate Grams
	Grams								
Fresh-pack, slices 1½ in. diam., ¼ in. thick, 2 slices	15	79	10	T	T	•	•	•	3
Sweet, gherkin, small, whole, about 2½ in. long, ¾ in. diam., 1 pickle	15	61	20	T	T	•	•	•	5
Pineapple:									
Raw, diced, 1 cup	155	85	80	1	T	•	•	•	21
Pineapple juice, unsweetened, canned, 1 cup	250	86	140	1	T	•	•	•	34
Pizza (cheese) baked, 4¾ in. sector; ⅛ of 12 in. diam. pie, 1 sector	60	45	145	6	4	1.7	1.5	.6	22
Plums:									
Raw, without pits: Japanese and hybrid (2⅛ in. diam., about 6½ per lb. with pits), 1 plum	66	87	30	T	T	•	•	•	8

Food									
Prune-type (1½ in. diam., about 15 per lb. with pits), 1 plum	28	79	20	T	T	•	•	•	6
Popcorn, popped:									
Plain, large kernel, 1 cup	6	4	25	1	1	T	.1	.2	5
With oil (coconut) and salt added, large kernel, 1 cup	9	3	40	1	2	1.5	.2	.2	5
Sugar coated, 1 cup	35	4	135	1	1	.5	.2	.2	5
Pork, cured, cooked:									
Ham, light cure, lean and fat, roasted (2 pieces, 4⅛ by 2¼ by ¼ in.), 3 oz.	85	54	245	18	19	6.8	7.9	1.7	0
Luncheon meat:									
Boiled ham, slice (8 per 8 oz. pkg.), 1 oz.	28	59	65	5	5	1.7	2.0	.4	0
Canned, spiced or unspiced: Slice, approx. 3 by 2 by ½ in., 1 slice	60	55	175	9	15	5.4	6.7	1.0	1
Chop, loin (cut 3 per lb. with bone), broiled: Lean and fat, 2¾ oz.	78	42	305	19	25	8.9	10.4	2.2	0

Foods, approximate measures, units and weight (edible part unless footnotes indicate otherwise)		Water Percent	Food Energy Calories	Protein Grams	Fat (Total) Grams	Saturated (Total) Grams	Unsaturated Oleic Grams	Linoleic Grams	Carbohydrate Grams
	Grams	Percent	Calories	Grams	Grams	Grams	Grams	Grams	Grams
Roast, oven cooked, no liquid added:									
Lean and fat (piece, 2½ by 2½ by ¾ in.), 3 oz.	85	46	310	21	24	8.7	10.2	2.2	0
Shoulder cut, simmered:									
Lean and fat (3 pieces, 2½ by 2½ by ¼ in.), 3 oz.	85	46	320	20	26	9.3	10.9	2.3	0
Pork link (16 per 1 lb. pkg.), cooked, 1 link	13	35	60	2	6	2.1	2.4	.5	T
Potato chips, 1¾ by 2½ in oval cross section, 10 chips	20	2	115	1	8	2.1	1.4	4.0	10
Potatoes, cooked:									
Baked, peeled after baking (about 2 per lb. raw), 1 potato	156	75	145	4	T	•	•	•	33
Boiled (about 3 per lb. raw):									
Peeled after boiling, 1 potato	137	80	105	3	T	•	•	•	23

	Weight (g)	Water (%)	Food energy (cal)	Protein (g)	Fat (g)	Saturated (g)	Unsaturated Oleic (g)	Unsaturated Linoleic (g)	Carbohydrate (g)
French-fried, strip, 2 to 3½ in. long:									
Prepared from raw, 10 strips	50	45	135	2	7	1.7	1.2	3.3	18
Hashed brown, prepared from frozen, 1 cup	155	56	345	3	18	4.6	3.2	9.0	45
Mashed, prepared from—Raw:									
Milk and butter added, 1 cup	210	80	195	4	9	5.6	2.3	.2	26
Potato salad, made with cooked salad dressing, 1 cup	250	76	250	7	7	2.0	2.7	1.3	41
Pretzels, made with enriched flour:									
Thin, twisted, 3¼ by 2¼ by ¼ in., 10 pretzels	60	5	235		3	—	—	—	46
Prune juice, canned or bottled, 1 cup	256	80	195	1	T	—	—	—	49
Prunes, dried: "softenized," with pits:									
Uncooked, 4 extra large or 5 large prunes	49		110	1	T	—	—	—	29
Cooked, unsweetened, all sizes, fruit and liquid, 1 cup	250		225			—	—	—	67
Puddings:									
From mix (chocolate) and milk:									
Regular (cooked), 1 cup	260	70	320			4.?		.2	59

Foods, approximate measures, units and weight (edible part unless footnotes indicate otherwise)		Water Percent	Food Energy Calories	Protein Grams	Fat (Total) Grams	Saturated (Total) Grams	Unsaturated Oleic Grams	Unsaturated Linoleic Grams	Carbohydrate Grams
	Grams								
Instant, 1 cup	260	69	325	8	7	3.6	2.2	.3	63
Pumpkin, canned, 1 cup	245	90	80	2	1	•	•	•	19
Radishes, raw (prepackaged) stem ends, rootlets cut off, 4 radishes	18	95	5	T	T				1
Raisins, seedless:									
Cup, not pressed down, 1 cup	145	18	420	4	T	•	•	•	112
Raspberries, red:									
Raw, capped, whole, 1 cup	123	84	70	1	1	•	•	•	17
Rhubarb, cooked, added sugar:									
From raw, 1 cup	270	63	380	1	T	•	•	•	97
Rice, white, enriched:									
Instant, ready-to-serve, hot, 1 cup	165	73	180	4	T	T	T	T	40
Long grain:									
Raw, 1 cup	185	12	670	12	1	.2	.2	.2	149
Cooked, served hot, 1 cup	205	73	225	4	T	.1	.1	.1	50

Rolls, enriched:

Commercial:

Brown-and-serve (12 per 12 oz. pkg), browned, 1 roll	26	27	85	2	2	.4	.7	.5	14
Cloverleaf or pan, 2½ in. diam., 2 in. high, 1 roll	28	31	85	2	2	.4	.6	.4	15
Frankfurter and hamburger (8 per 11½ oz. pkg), 1 roll	40	31	120	3	2	.5	.8	.6	21
Hard, 3¾ in. diam., 2 in. high, 1 roll	50	25	155	5	2	.4	.6	.5	30
Hoagie or submarine, 11½ by 3 by 2½ in., 1 roll	135	31	390	12	4	.9	1.4	1.4	75

Salad dressings:

Commercial:

Blue cheese: Regular, 1 tbsp.	15	32	75	1	8	1.6	1.7	3.8	1
Low calorie (5 Cal. per tsp.), 1 tbsp.	16	84	10	T	1	.5	.3	T	1
French: Regular, 1 tbsp.	16	39	65	T	6	1.1	1.3	3.2	3
Low calorie (5 Cal. per tsp.), 1 tbsp.	16	77	15	T	1	.1	.1	.4	2
Italian: Regular, 1 tbsp.	15	28	85	T	9	1.6	1.9	4.7	1

Foods, approximate measures, units and weight (edible part unless footnotes indicate otherwise)		Water	Food Energy	Protein	Fat (Total)	Saturated (Total)	Unsaturated Oleic	Linoleic	Carbohydrate
	Grams	Percent	Calories	Grams	Grams	Grams	Grams	Grams	Grams
Low calorie (2 Cal. per tsp.), 1 tbsp.	15	90	10	T	1	.1	.1	.4	T
Mayonnaise, 1 tbsp.	14	15	100	T	11	2.0	2.4	5.6	T
Mayonnaise type:									
Regular, 1 tbsp.	15	41	65	T	6	1.1	1.4	3.2	2
Low calorie (8 Cal. per tsp.), 1 tbsp.	16	81	20	T	2	.4	1.8	4.1	1
Tartar sauce, regular, 1 tbsp.	14	34	75	T	8	1.5	1.8	4.1	1
Thousand Island:									
Regular, 1 tbsp.	16	32	80	T	8	1.4	1.7	4.0	2
Low calorie (10 Cal. per tsp.), 1 tbsp.	15	68	25	T	2	.4	.4	1.0	2
Salami:									
Dry type, slice (12 per 4 oz. pkg.), 1 slice	10	30	45	2	4	1.6	1.6	.1	T
Cooked type, slice (8 per 8 oz. pkg.), 1 slice	28	51	90	5	7	3.1	3.0	.1	T

	Grams	Water (%)	Food energy	Protein	Fat	Saturated	Unsaturated (oleic)	Unsaturated (linoleic)	Carbohydrate
Salmon, pink, canned, solids and liquid, 3 oz.	85	71	120	17	5	.9	.8	.1	0
Sardines, Atlantic, canned in oil, drained solids, 3 oz.	85	62	175	20	9	3.0	2.5	.5	0
Sauerkraut, canned, solids and liquid, 1 cup	235	93	40	2	T	•	•	•	9
Scallops, frozen, breaded, fried, reheated, 6 scallops	90	60	175	16	8	•	•	•	9
Shad, baked with butter or margarine, bacon, 3 oz.	85	64	170	20	10	•	•	•	0
Shrimp:									
Canned meat, 3 oz.	85	70	100	21	1	.1	.1	T	1
French fried, 3 oz.	85	57	190	17	9	2.3	3.7	2.0	9
Soups:									
Canned, condensed:									
Prepared with equal volume of milk:									
Cream of chicken, 1 cup	245	85	180	7	10	4.2	3.6	1.3	15
Cream of mushroom, 1 cup	245	83	215	7	14	5.4	2.9	4.6	16
Tomato, 1 cup	250	84	175	7	7	3.4	1.7	1.0	23
Prepared with equal volume of water:									
Bean with pork, 1 cup	250	84	170	8	6	1.2	1.8	2.4	22

Foods, approximate measures, units and weight (edible part unless footnotes indicate otherwise)		Water Percent	Food Energy Calories	Protein Grams	Fat (Total) Grams	Saturated (Total) Grams	Unsaturated Oleic Grams	Linoleic Grams	Carbohydrate Grams
	Grams	Percent	Calories	Grams	Grams	Grams	Grams	Grams	Grams
Beef broth, bouillon, consomme, 1 cup	240	96	30	5	0	0	0	0	3
Beef noodle, 1 cup	240	93	65	4	3	.6	.7	.8	7
Clam chowder, Manhattan type, (with tomatoes, without milk), 1 cup	245	92	80	2	3	.5	.4	1.3	12
Cream of chicken, 1 cup	240	92	95	3	6	1.6	2.3	1.1	8
Cream of mushroom, 1 cup	240	90	135	2	10	2.6	1.7	4.5	10
Minestrone, 1 cup	245	90	105	5	3	.7	.9	1.3	14
Split pea, 1 cup	245	85	145	9	3	1.1	1.2	.4	21
Tomato, 1 cup	245	91	90	2	3	.5	.5	1.0	16
Vegetable beef, 1 cup	245	92	80	5	2	•	•	•	10
Vegetarian, 1 cup	245	92	80	2	2	•	•	•	13
Dehydrated: Bouillon cube, ½ in., 1 cube	4	4	5	1	T	•	•	•	T
Mixes: Unprepared: Onion, 1½ oz. pkg.	43	3	150	6	5	1.1	2.3	1.0	23

		Water	Food energy	Protein	Fat	Saturated	Oleic	Linoleic	Carbohydrate
	(g)	(%)	(cal.)	(g)	(g)				(g)
Prepared with water:									
Chicken noodle, 1 cup	240	95	55	2	1	••	••	••	8
Onion, 1 cup	240	96	35	1	1	••	••	••	6
Tomato vegetable with noodles, 1 cup	240	93	65	1	1	•	•	•	12
Spaghetti, enriched, cooked:									
Firm stage, "al dente," served hot, 1 cup	130	64	190	7	1	••	••	••	39
Tender stage, served hot, 1 cup	140	73	155	5	1	••	••	••	32
Spaghetti (enriched) in tomato sauce with cheese:									
From home recipe, 1 cup	250	77	260	9	9	2.0	5.4	.7	37
Spaghetti (enriched) with meat balls and tomato sauce:									
From home recipe, 1 cup	248	70	330	19	12	3.3	6.3	.9	39
Spinach:									
Raw, chopped, 1 cup	55	91	15	2	T	•	•	•	2
Cooked, drained:									
From raw, 1 cup	180	92	40	5	1	•	•	•	6
Squash, cooked:									
Summer (all varieties), diced, drained, 1 cup	210	96	30	2	T	•	•	•	7
Winter (all varieties), baked, mashed, 1 cup	205	81	130	4	1	•	•	•	32

Foods, approximate measures, units and weight (edible part unless footnotes indicate otherwise)		Water	Food Energy	Protein	Fat (Total)	Saturated (Total)	Unsaturated Oleic	Linoleic	Carbohydrate
	Grams	Percent	Calories	Grams	Grams	Grams	Grams	Grams	Grams
Strawberries:									
Raw, whole berries, capped, 1 cup	149	90	55	1	1	•	•	•	13
Frozen, sweetened:									
Sliced, 10 oz. container, 1 container	284	71	310	1	1	•	•	•	79
Whole, 1 lb. container (about 1¾ cups), 1 container	454	76	415	2	1	•	•	•	107
Sunflower seeds, dry, hulled, 1 cup	145	5	810	35	69	8.2	13.7	43.2	29
Sugars:									
Brown, pressed down, 1 cup	220	2	820	0	0	0	0	0	212
White:									
Granulated, 1 cup	200	1	770	0	0	0	0	0	199
Sweet potatoes:									
Cooked (raw, 5 by 2 in.; about 2½ per lb.):									
Baked in skin, peeled, 1 potato	114	64	160	2	1	•	•	•	37

Food, approximate measure	Grams	Water (%)	Calories	Protein (g)	Fat (g)	Saturated (g)	Unsaturated, Oleic (g)	Unsaturated, Linoleic (g)	Carbohydrate (g)
Candied, 2½ by 2 in. piece, 1 potato	105	60	175	1	3	2.0	.8	.1	36
Tangerine, raw, 2⅜ in. diam., size 176, without peel (about 4 per lb. with peels and seeds), 1 tangerine	86	87	40	1	T	•	•	•	10
Tangerine juice, canned, sweetened, 1 cup	249	87	125	1	T	•	•	•	30
Tomato catsup, 1 tbsp.	15	69	15	T	T	•	•	•	4
Tomatoes: Raw, 2⅗ in. diam. (3 per 12 oz. pkg.), 1 tomato	135	94	25	1	T	•	•	•	6
Tomato juice, canned: Cup, 1 cup	243	94	45	2	T	•	•	•	10
Tuna, canned in oil, drained solids, 3 oz.	85	61	170	24	7	1.7	1.7	.7	0
Tuna salad, 1 cup	205	70	350	30	22	4.3	6.3	6.7	7
Turkey, roasted, flesh without skin: Dark meat, piece, 2½ by 1⅝ by ¼ in., 4 pieces	85	61	175	26	7	2.1	1.5	1.5	0
Light meat, piece, 4 by 2 by ¼ in., 2 pieces	85	62	150	28	3	.9	.6	.7	0

Foods, approximate measures, units and weight (edible part unless footnotes indicate otherwise)		Water	Food Energy	Protein	Fat (Total)	Saturated (Total)	Unsaturated Oleic	Linoleic	Carbohydrate
	Grams	Percent	Calories	Grams	Grams	Grams	Grams	Grams	Grams
Turnip greens, cooked, drained:									
From raw (leaves and stems), 1 cup	145	94	30	3	T	(•)	(•)	(•)	5
Turnips, cooked, diced, 1 cup	155	94	35	1	T	(•)	(•)	(•)	8
Veal, medium fat, cooked, bone removed:									
Cutlet (4⅛ by 2¼ by ½ in.), braised or broiled, 3 oz.	85	60	185	23	9	4.0	3.4	.4	0
Rib (2 pieces, 4⅛ by 2¼ by ¼ in.), roasted, 3 oz.	85	55	230	23	14	6.1	5.1	.6	0
Vegetables, mixed, frozen, cooked, 1 cup	182	83	115	6	1	(•)	(•)	(•)	24
Vienna sausage (7 per 4 oz. can), 1 sausage	16	63	40	2	3	1.2	1.4	.2	T
Vinegar, cider, 1 tbsp.	15	94	T	T	0	0	0	0	1
Waffles, made with enriched flour, 7 in diam.:									
From home recipe, 1 waffle	75	41	210	7	7	2.3	2.8	1.4	28

Food									
From mix, egg and milk added, 1 waffle	75	42	205	7	8	2.8	2.9	1.2	27
Walnuts:									
Black:									
Chopped or broken kernels, 1 cup	125	3	785	26	74	6.3	13.3	45.7	19
Ground (finely), 1 cup	80	3	500	16	47	4.0	8.5	29.2	12
Watermelon, raw, 4 by 8 in. wedge with rind and seeds (1/16 of 32 2/3 lb. melon, 10 by 16 in.), 1 wedge with, rind and seeds	926	93	110	2	1	•	•	•	27
Wheat flours:									
All-purpose or family flour, enriched:									
Sifted, spooned, 1 cup	115	12	420	12	1	.2	.1	.5	88
Unsifted, spooned, 1 cup	125	12	455	13	1	.2	.1	.5	95
Cake or pastry flour, enriched, sifted, spooned, 1 cup	96	12	350	7	1	.1	.1	.3	76
Self-rising, enriched, unsifted, spooned, 1 cup	125	12	440	12	1	.2	.1	.5	93
Whole wheat, from hard wheats, stirred, 1 cup	120	12	400	16	2	.4	.2	1.0	85

Foods, approximate measures, units and weight (edible part unless footnotes indicate otherwise)		Water	Food Energy	Protein	Fat (Total)	Saturated (Total)	Unsaturated Oleic	Linoleic	Carbohydrate
	Grams	Percent	Calories	Grams	Grams	Grams	Grams	Grams	Grams
White sauce, medium, with enriched flour, 1 cup	250	73	405	10	31	19.3	7.8	.8	22
Wines:									
Dessert, 3½ fl. oz. glass	103	77	140	T	0	0	0	0	8
Table, 3½ fl. oz. glass	102	86	85	T	0	0	0	0	4
Yogurt:									
With added milk solids:									
Made with lowfat milk:									
Fruit flavored, 1 container, net wt. 8 oz.	227	75	230	10	3	1.8	.6	.1	42
Plain, 1 container, net wt. 8 oz.	227	85	145	12	4	2.3	.8	.1	16
Made with nonfat milk, 1 container, net wt. 8 oz.	227	85	125	13	T	.3	.1	T	17
Without added milk solids:									
Made with whole milk, 1 container, net wt. 8 oz.	227	88	140	8	7	4.8	1.7	.1	11

Appendix 1

NUTRITIVE VALUES OF THE EDIBLE PART OF FOODS

(A dot ● denotes lack of reliable data for a constituent
believed to be present in measurable amount;
the letter T indicates that a trace of the constituent in question is present.)

Vitamins and Minerals in Indicated Quantity

Foods, approximate measures, units and weight (edible part unless footnotes indicate otherwise)	Calcium Milli- grams	Phosphorus Milli- grams	Iron Milli- grams	Potassium Milli- grams	Vitamin A Value Internat'l. units	Thiamin Milli- grams	Ribo- flavin Milli- grams	Niacin Milli- grams	Ascorbic Acid Milli- grams
Almonds, shelled Chopped (about 130 almonds), 1 cup	304	655	6.1	1,005	0	.31	1.20	4.6	T
Apples, raw, unpeeled, 3¼ in. diam. (about 2 per lb. with cores), 1 apple	15	21	.6	233	190	.06	.04	.2	8

Foods, approximate measures, units and weight (edible part unless footnotes indicate otherwise)	Calcium	Phosphorus	Iron	Potassium	Vitamin A Value	Thiamin	Riboflavin	Niacin	Ascorbic Acid
	Milli-grams	Milli-grams	Milli-grams	Milli-grams	Internat'l. units	Milli-grams	Milli-grams	Milli-grams	Milli-grams
Apricots: Raw, without pits (about 12 per lb. with pits), 3 apricots	18	25	.5	301	2,890	.03	.04	.6	11
Asparagus, green: Cooked, drained: Spears, ½-in. diam. at base: From raw, 4 spears	13	30	.4	110	540	.10	.11	.8	16
Bacon, (20 slices per lb. raw), broiled or fried, crisp, 2 slices	2	34	.5	35	0	.08	.05	.8	•
Bagel, Egg, 3-in. diam., 1 bagel	9	43	1.2	41	30	.14	.10	1.2	0
Banana without peel (about 2½ per lb. with peel), 1 banana	10	31	.8	440	230	.06	.07	.8	12
Beans: Babys Limas, 1 cup	63	227	4.7	709	400	.16	.09	2.2	22

Green:								
From raw (cuts and French style), 1 cup	63	46	.8	189	680	.09	.11	.6	15
Yellow or wax:								
From raw (cuts and French style), 1 cup	63	46	.8	189	290	.09	.11	.6	16
Bean sprouts (mung):								
Raw, 1 cup	20	67	1.4	234	20	.14	.14	.8	20
Beef, cooked:								
Cuts braised, simmered or pot roasted:								
Lean and fat (piece, 2½ by 2½ by ¾ in.), 3 oz.	10.	114	2.9	184	30	.04	.18	3.6	•
Ground Beef, broiled:								
Lean with 10% fat, 3 oz. or patty 3 by ⅝ in.	10	196	3.0	261	20	.08	.20	5.1	•
Roast, oven cooked, no liquid added:								
Relatively fat, such as rib:								
Lean and fat (2 pieces, 4⅛ by 2¼ by ¼ in.), 3 oz.	8	158	2.2	189	70	.05	.13	3.1	•

Foods, approximate measures, units and weight (edible part unless footnotes indicate otherwise)	Calcium	Phosphorus	Iron	Potassium	Vitamin A Value	Thiamin	Riboflavin	Niacin	Ascorbic Acid
	Milligrams	Milligrams	Milligrams	Milligrams	International units	Milligrams	Milligrams	Milligrams	Milligrams
Roast, oven cooked, no liquid added:									
Relatively lean, such as heel of round:									
Lean and fat (2 pieces), 4⅛ by 2¼ by ¼ in., 3 oz.	11	208	3.2	279	10	.06	.19	4.5	•
Steak:									
Relatively fat, sirloin, broiled:									
Lean and fat (piece, 2½ by ¾ in.), 3 oz.	9	162	2.5	220	50	.05	.15	4.0	•
Relatively lean, round, braised:									
Lean and fat (piece, 4⅛ by 2¼ by ½ in., 3 oz.	10	213	3.0	272	20	.07	.19	4.8	•
Beer, 12 fl. oz.	18	108	T	90	•	.01	.11	2.2	•
Beets:									
Whole beets, 2-in. diam., 2 beets	14	23	.5	208	20	.03	.04	.3	6

Food									
Biscuits, baking powder, 2-in. diam. (enriched flour, vegetable shortening): From mix, 1 biscuit	19	65	.6	32	T	.09	.08	.8	T
Blackeyed peas, dry, cooked (with residual cooking liquid), 1 cup	43	238	3.3	573	30	.40	.10	1.0	•
Blackberries, raw, 1 cup	46	27	1.3	245	290	.04	.06	.6	30
Blueberries, raw, 1 cup	22	19	1.5	117	150	.04	.09	.7	20
Bluefish, baked with butter or margarine, 3 oz.	25	244	.6	•	40	.09	.08	1.6	•
Bologna, slice (8 per 8-oz. pkg.), 1 slice	2	36	.5	65	•	.05	.06	.7	•
Braunschweiger, slice (6 per 6-oz. pkg.), 1 slice	3	69	1.7	•	1,850	.05	.41	2.3	•
Brazil nuts, shelled (6-8 large kernels), 1 oz.	53	196	1.0	203	T	.27	.03	.5	•
Breads Cracked-wheat bread (¾ enriched wheat flour, ¼ cracked wheat): Slice (18 per loaf), 1 slice	22	32	.5	34	T	.08	.06	.8	T

Foods, approximate measures, units and weight (edible part unless footnotes indicate otherwise)	Calcium	Phosphorus	Iron	Potassium	Vitamin A Value	Thiamin	Riboflavin	Niacin	Ascorbic Acid
	Milligrams	Milligrams	Milligrams	Milligrams	International units	Milligrams	Milligrams	Milligrams	Milligrams
French or Vienna bread, enriched: Slice:									
French (5 by 2½ by 1 in.), 1 slice	15	30	.8	32	T	.14	.08	1.2	T
Vienna (4¾ by 4 by ½ in.), 1 slice	11	21	.6	23	T	.10	.06	.8	T
Italian bread enriched: Slice, 4½ by 3¼ by 1 in., 1 slice	5	23	.7	22	0	.12	.07	1.0	0
Raisin bread, enriched: Slice (18 per loaf), 1 slice	18	22	.6	58	T	.09	.06	.6	T
Rye Bread: American, light (⅔ enriched wheat flour, ⅓ rye flour): Slice (4¾ by 3¾ by 7/16 in.), 1 slice	19	37	.5	36	0	.07	.05	.7	0

Food									
Pumpernickel (⅔ rye flour, ⅓ enriched wheat flour):									
Slice (5 by 4 by ⅜ in.), 1 slice	27	73	.8	145	0	.09	.07	.6	0
White Bread, enriched:									
Soft-crumb type:									
Slice (18 per loaf), 1 slice	21	24	.6	26	T	.10	.06	.8	T
Slice, toasted, 1 slice	21	24	.6	26	T	.08	.06	.8	T
Firm-crumb type:									
Slice (20 per loaf), 1 slice	22	23	.6	28	T	.09	.06	.8	T
Slice, toasted, 1 slice	22	23	.6	28	T	.07	.06	.8	T
Whole-wheat bread:									
Soft-crumb type:									
Slice (16 per loaf), 1 slice	24	71	.8	72	T	.09	.03	.8	T
Slice, toasted, 1 slice	24	71	.8	72	T	.07	.03	.8	T
Firm-crumb type:									
Slice (18 per loaf), 1 slice	25	57	.8	68	T	.06	.03	.7	T
Slice, toasted, 1 slice	25	57	.8	68	T	.05	.04	.7	T
Breakfast cereals:									
Hot type, cooked:									
Farina, quick-cooking, enriched, 1 cup	147	113	(*)	25	0	.12	.07	1.0	0
Oatmeal or rolled oats, 1 cup	22	137	1.4	146	0	.19	.05	.2	0
Wheat, whole-meal, 1 cup	17	127	1.2	118	0	.15	.05	1.5	0

(*)Value may range from less than 1 mg. to about 8 mg. depending on the brand. Consult the label.

Foods, approximate measures, units and weight (edible part unless footnotes indicate otherwise)	Calcium	Phosphorus	Iron	Potassium	Vitamin A Value	Thiamin	Ribo-flavin	Niacin	Ascorbic Acid
	Milli-grams	Milli-grams	Milli-grams	Milli-grams	Internat'l. units	Milli-grams	Milli-grams	Milli-grams	Milli-grams
Ready-to-eat:									
Bran flakes (40% bran), added sugar, salt, iron, vitamins, 1 cup	19	125	15.6	137	1,650	.41	.49	4.1	12
Corn flakes:									
Plain, added sugar, salt, iron, vitamins, 1 cup	(**)	9	.6	30	1,180	.29	.35	2.9	9
Sugar-coated, added salt, iron, vitamins, 1 cup	1	10	1.0	27	1,880	.46	.56	4.6	14
Corn, puffed, plain, added sugar, salt, iron, vitamins, 1 cup	4	18	2.3	•	940	.23	.28	2.3	7
Corn, shredded, added sugar, salt, iron, thiamin, niacin, 1 cup	1	10	.6	•	0	.11	.05	.5	0
Oats, puffed, added sugar, salt, minerals, vitamins, 1 cup	44	102	2.9	•	1,180	.29	.35	2.9	9

Rice, puffed:									
Plain, added iron, thiamin, niacin, 1 cup	3	14	.3	15	0	.07	.01	.7	0
Wheat flakes, added sugar, salt, iron, vitamins, 1 cup	12	83	(**)	81	1,410	.35	.42	3.5	11
Wheat, puffed:									
Plain, added iron, thiamin, niacin, 1 cup	4	48	.6	51	0	.08	.03	1.2	0
Presweetened, added salt, iron, vitamins, 1 cup	7	52	1.6	63	1,680	.50	.57	6.7	20
Wheat, shredded, plain, 1 oblong biscuit or ½ cup spoon-size biscuits	11	97	.9	87	0	.06	.03	1.1	0
Wheat germ without salt and sugar, toasted, 1 tbsp.	3	70	.5	57	10	.11	.05	.3	1
Broccoli:									
From stalk, medium size, 1 stalk	158	112	1.4	481	4,500	.16	.36	1.4	162
Brussel sprouts, cooked, drained: From raw, 7-8 sprouts (1¼ to 1½ in. diam.), 1 cup	50	112	1.7	423	810	.12	.22	1.2	135
Butter:									
Tablespoon (about ⅛ stick), 1 tbsp.	3	3	T	4	430	T	T	T	0

(**)Value varies with the brand. Consult the label.

Foods, approximate measures, units and weight (edible part unless footnotes indicate otherwise)	Calcium	Phosphorus	Iron	Potassium	Vitamin A Value	Thiamin	Riboflavin	Niacin	Ascorbic Acid
	Milligrams	Milligrams	Milligrams	Milligrams	International units	Milligrams	Milligrams	Milligrams	Milligrams
Whipped (6 sticks or two 8-oz. containers per lb.): Tablespoon (about ⅛ stick), 1 tbsp.	2	2	T	2	290	T	T	T	0
Cabbage:									
Raw, coarsely shredded or sliced, 1 cup	34	20	.3	163	90	.04	.04	.02	33
Cooked, drained, 1 cup	64	29	.4	236	190	.06	.06	.4	48
Red, raw, coarsely shredded or sliced, 1 cup	29	25	.6	188	30	.06	.04	.3	43
Savory, raw, coarsely shredded or sliced, 1 cup	47	38	.6	188	140	.04	.06	.2	39
Cakes made from cake mixes with enriched flour: Angelfood: Whole cake (9¾ in. diam. tube cake), 1 cake	603	756	2.5	381	0	.37	.95	3.6	0

Coffeecake: Whole cake (7¾ by 5⅝ by 1¼ in.), 1 cake	262	748	6.9	469	690	.82	.91	7.7	1
Cupcakes, made with egg, milk, 2½ in. diam.: Without icing, 1 cupcake	40	59	.3	21	40	.05	.05	.4	T
With chocolate icing, 1 cupcake	47	71	.4	42	60	.05	.05	.4	T
Devil's food with chocolate icing: Whole, 2 layer cake (8 or 9 in. diam.), 1 cake	653	1,162	16.6	1,439	1,660	1.06	1.65	10.1	1
Cupcake, 2½ in. diam, 1 cupcake	21	37	.5	46	50	.03	.05	.3	T
Gingerbread: Whole cake (8 in. square), 1 cake	513	570	8.6	1,562	T	.84	1.00	7.4	T
White, 2 layer with chocolate icing: Whole cake (8 or 9 in. diam.), 1 cake	1,129	2,041	11.4	1,322	680	1.50	1.77	12.5	2
Yellow, 2 layer with chocolate icing: Whole cake (8 or 9 in. diam.), 1 cake	1,008	2,017	12.2	1,208	1,550	1.24	1.67	10.6	2

Foods, approximate measures, units and weight (edible part unless footnotes indicate otherwise)	Calcium	Phosphorus	Iron	Potassium	Vitamin A Value	Thiamin	Riboflavin	Niacin	Ascorbic Acid
	Milligrams	Milligrams	Milligrams	Milligrams	Internat'l. units	Milligrams	Milligrams	Milligrams	Milligrams
Cantaloupe, orange-fleshed (with rind and seed cavity, 5 in. diam., 2⅓ lb.), ½ melon with rind	38	44	1.1	682	9,240	.11	.08	1.6	90
Carrots: Raw, without crowns and tips, scraped: Whole, 7½ by 1⅛ in. or strips, 2½ to 3 in. long, 1 carrot or 18 strips	27	26	.5	246	7,930	.04	.04	.4	6
Cooked (crosswise cuts), drained, 1 cup	51	48	.9	344	16,280	.08	.08	.8	9
Cashew nuts, roasted in oil, 1 cup	53	522	5.3	650	140	.60	.35	2.5	•
Cauliflower: Cooked, from raw (flower buds), 1 cup	26	53	.9	258	80	.11	.10	.8	69

Food									
Celery, Pascal type, raw:									
Stalk, larger outer, 8 by 1½ in. at root end, 1 stalk	16	11	.1	136	110	.01	.01	.1	4
Cheese:									
Natural:									
Blue, 1 oz.	150	110	.1	73	200	.01	.11	.3	0
Camembert (3 wedges per 4 oz. container), 1 wedge	147	132	.1	71	350	.01	.19	.2	0
Cheddar:									
Cut pieces, 1 oz.	204	145	.2	28	300	.01	.11	T	0
Cottage (curd not pressed down):									
Creamed (cottage cheese, 4% fat):									
Large curd, 1 cup	135	297	.3	190	370	.05	.37	.3	T
Small curd, 1 cup	126	277	.3	177	340	.04	.34	.3	T
Low fat (1%), 1 cup	138	302	.3	193	80	.05	.37	.3	T
Cream, 1 oz.	23	30	.3	34	400	T	.06	T	0
Mozzarella, made with:									
Whole milk, 1 oz.	163	117	.1	21	260	T	.08	T	0
Part skim milk, 1 oz.	207	149	.1	27	180	.01	.10	T	0
Parmesan, grated:									
Tablespoon, 1 tbsp.	69	40	T	5	40	T	.02	T	0

273

Foods, approximate measures, units and weight (edible part unless footnotes indicate otherwise)	Calcium	Phosphorus	Iron	Potassium	Vitamin A Value	Thiamin	Riboflavin	Niacin	Ascorbic Acid
	Milligrams	Milligrams	Milligrams	Milligrams	International units	Milligrams	Milligrams	Milligrams	Milligrams
Provolone, 1 oz.	214	141	.1	39	230	.01	.09	T	0
Ricotta, made with:									
Whole milk, 1 cup	509	389	.9	257	1,210	.03	.48	.3	0
Part skim milk, 1 cup	669	449	1.1	308	1,060	.05	.46	.2	0
Romano, 1 oz.	302	215	•	•	160	•	.11	T	0
Swiss, 1 oz.	272	171	T	31	240	.01	.10	T	0
Pasteurized processed cheese:									
American, 1 oz.	174	211	.1	46	340	.01	.10	T	0
Swiss, 1 oz.	219	216	.2	61	230	T	.08	T	0
Cherries:									
Sweet, raw, without pits and stems, 10 cherries	15	13	.3	129	70	.03	.04	.3	7
Chicken, cooked:									
Breast, fried, bones removed, ½ breast (3⅓ oz. with bones), 2¾ oz.	9	218	1.3	•	70	.04	.17	11.6	•

Food									
Drumstick, fried, bones removed (2 oz. with bones), 13 oz.	6	89	.9	•	50	.03	.15	2.7	•
Half broiler, broiled, bones removed (10½ oz. with bones), 6¼ oz.	16	355	3.0	483	160	.09	.34	15.5	•
Chili con carne with beans, canned, 1 cup	82	321	4.3	594	150	.08	.18	3.3	•
Chocolate: Bitter or baking, 1 oz.	22	109	1.9	235	20	.01	.07	.4	0
Semisweet, see Candy, chocolate.									
Chocolate milk (commercial): Regular, 1 cup	280	251	.6	417	300	.09	.41	.3	2
Lowfat (1%), 1 cup	287	257	.6	426	500	.10	.40	.2	2
Clams: Raw, meat only, 3 oz.	59	138	5.2	154	90	.08	.15	1.1	8
Coconut meat, fresh: Shredded or grated, not pressed down, 1 cup	10	76	1.4	205	0	.04	.02	.4	2
Cola drink, 12 fl. oz.	•	•	•	•	0	0	0	0	0

Foods, approximate measures, units and weight (edible part unless footnotes indicate otherwise)	Calcium	Phosphorus	Iron	Potassium	Vitamin A Value	Thiamin	Riboflavin	Niacin	Ascorbic Acid
	Milligrams	Milligrams	Milligrams	Milligrams	International units	Milligrams	Milligrams	Milligrams	Milligrams
Cookies made with enriched flour:									
Brownies with nuts:									
Home-prepared, 1¾ by 1¾ by ⅞ in.:									
From home recipe, 1 brownie	8	30	.4	38	40	.04	.03	.2	T
From commercial recipe, 1 brownie	9	27	.4	34	20	.03	.02	.2	T
Chocolate Chip:									
Commercial, 2¼ in. diam., ⅛ in. thick, 4 cookies	16	48	1.0	56	50	.10	.17	.9	T
From home recipe, 2⅓ in. diam., 4 cookies	14	40	.8	47	40	.06	.06	.5	T
Gingersnaps, 2 in. diam., ¼ in. thick, 4 cookies	20	13	.7	129	20	.08	.06	.7	0
Macaroons, 2¾ in. diam., ¼ in. thick, 2 cookies	10	32	.3	176	0	.02	.06	.2	0

Food								
Oatmeal with raisins, 2⅝ in. diam., ¼ in. thick, 4 cookies	11	53	1.4	192	30	.15	.10	1.0	T
Sandwich type (chocolate or vanilla), 1¾ in. diam., ⅜ in. thick, 4 cookies	10	96	.7	15	0	.06	.10	.7	0
Vanilla Wafers, 1¾ in. diam., ¼ in. thick, 10 cookies	16	25	.6	29	50	.10	.09	.8	0
Corn, sweet: Cooked, drained: From raw, ear 5 by 1¾ in., 1 ear	2	69	.5	151	310	.09	.08	1.1	7
Crabmeat (white or king), canned, not pressed down, 1 cup	61	246	1.1	149	•	.11	.11	2.6	•
Crackers: Graham, plain, 2½ in. square, 2 crackers	6	21	.5	55	0	.02	.08	.5	0
Rye wafers, whole-grain, 1⅞ by 3½ in., 2 wafers	7	50	.5	78	0	.04	.03	.2	0
Saltines, made with enriched flour, 4 crackers or 1 packet	2	10	.5	13	0	.05	.05	.4	0
Cranberry juice cocktail, bottled, sweetened, 1 cup	13	8	.8	25	T	.03	.03	.1	81

Foods, approximate measures, units and weight (edible part unless footnotes indicate otherwise)	Calcium Milli-grams	Phosphorus Milli-grams	Iron Milli-grams	Potassium Milli-grams	Vitamin A Value Internat'l. units	Thiamin Milli-grams	Ribo-flavin Milli-grams	Niacin Milli-grams	Ascorbic Acid Milli-grams
Cranberry sauce, sweetened, canned, strained, 1 cup	17	11	.6	83	60	.03	.03	.1	6
Cream products, imitation (made with vegetable fat):									
Sweet:									
Creamers:									
Liquid (frozen), 1 cup	23	157	.1	467	220	0	0	0	0
Powdered, 1 cup	21	397	.1	763	190	0	.16	0	0
Whipped topping:									
Frozen, 1 cup	5	6	.1	14	650	0	0	0	0
Pressurized, 1 cup	4	13	T	13	330	0	0	0	0
Cream, sour, 1 cup	268	195	.1	331	1,820	.08	.34	.2	2
Cream, sweet:									
Half-and-Half (cream and milk), 1 cup	254	230	.2	314	260	.08	.36	.2	2
Light, coffee, or table, 1 cup	231	192	.1	292	1,730	.08	.36	.1	2

Food									
Whipped, unwhipped (volume about double when whipped):									
Light, 1 cup	166	146	.1	231	2,690	.06	.30	.1	1
Heavy, 1 cup	154	149	.1	179	3,500	.05	.26	.1	1
Whipped topping (pressurized), 1 cup	61	54	T	88	550	.02	.04	T	0
Cucumber slices, ⅛ in. thick (large, 2⅛ in. diam.; small, 1¾ in. diam.):									
With peel, 6 large or 8 small slices	7	8	.3	45	70	.01	.01	.1	3
Custard, baked, 1 cup	297	310	1.1	387	930	.11	.50	.3	1
Dates:									
Whole, without pits, 10 dates	47	50	2.4	518	40	.07	.08	1.8	0
Doughnuts, made with enriched flour:									
Cake type, plain, 2½ in. diam., 1 in. high, 1 doughnut	10	48	.4	23	20	.05	.05	.4	T
Eggnog (commercial), 1 cup	330	278	.5	420	890	.09	.48	.3	4
Eggs, large (24 oz. per dozen):									
Cooked:									
Fried in butter, 1 egg	26	80	.9	58	290	.03	.13	T	0

279

Foods, approximate measures, units and weight (edible part unless footnotes indicate otherwise)	Calcium	Phosphorus	Iron	Potassium	Vitamin A Value	Thiamin	Ribo-flavin	Niacin	Ascorbic Acid
	Milli-grams	Milli-grams	Milli-grams	Milli-grams	Internat'l. units	Milli-grams	Milli-grams	Milli-grams	Milli-grams
Hard-cooked, shell removed, 1 egg	28	90	1.0	65	260	.04	.14	T	0
Poached, 1 egg	28	90	1.0	65	260	.04	.13	T	0
Scrambled (milk added) in butter, Also omelet, 1 egg	47	97	.9	85	310	.04	.16	T	0
Endive, curly (including escarole), raw, small pieces, 1 cup	41	27	.9	147	1,650	.04	.07	.3	5
Fats, cooking (vegetable shortenings), 1 cup	0	0	0	0	••	0	0	0	0
1 tbsp.	0	0	0	0	••	0	0	0	0
Filberts (hazelnuts), chopped (about 80 kernels), 1 cup	240	388	3.9	8.0	•	.53	•	1.0	T
Fish sticks, breaded, cooked, frozen (stick, 4 by 1 by ½ in.), 1 fish stick or 1 oz.	3	47	.1	•	0	.01	.02	.5	•

Food									
Frankfurter (8 per 1 lb. pkg.), cooked (reheated), 1 frankfurter	3	57	.8	•	•	.08	.11	1.4	•
Fruit cocktail, canned, in heavy syrup, 1 cup	23	31	1.0	411	360	.05	.03	1.0	5
Fruit-flavored sodas and Tom Collins mixer, 12 fl. oz.	•	•	•	•	0	0	0	0	0
Gelatin dessert prepared with gelatin dessert powder and water, 1 cup	•	•	•	•	0	0	0	0	0
Ginger ale, 12 fl. oz.	•	•	•	•	0	0	0	0	0
Grape drink, canned, 1 cup	8	10	.3	88	•	.03	.03	.3	(*)
Grapefruit juice: Canned, white: Unsweetened, 1 cup	20	35	1.0	400	20	.07	.05	.5	84
Frozen, concentrate, unsweetened: Diluted with 3 parts water by volume, 1 cup	25	42	.2	420	20	.10	.04	.5	95

(*)For products with added thiamin and riboflavin but without added ascorbic acid, values in milligrams would be 0.60 for thiamin, 0.80 for riboflavin, and trace for ascorbic acid.
For products with ascorbic acid added, value varies with the brand, Consult the label.

Foods, approximate measures, units and weight (edible part unless footnotes indicate otherwise)	Calcium Milligrams	Phosphorus Milligrams	Iron Milligrams	Potassium Milligrams	Vitamin A Value International units	Thiamin Milligrams	Riboflavin Milligrams	Niacin Milligrams	Ascorbic Acid Milligrams
Grapefruit: Raw, medium, 3¾ in. diam. (about 1 lb. 1 oz.).: White, ½ grapefruit with peel	19	19	.5	159	10	.05	.02	.2	44
Grape juice: Canned or bottled, 1 cup	28	30	.8	293	•	.10	.05	.5	T
Frozen concentrate, sweetened: Diluted with 3 parts water by volume, 1 cup	8	10	.3	85	10	.05	.08	.5	10
Grapes, European type (adherent skin) raw: Thompson Seedless, 10 grapes	6	10	.2	87	50	.03	.02	.2	2
Tokay and Emperor seeded types, 10 grapes	7	11	.2	99	60	.03	.02	.2	2
Haddock, breaded, fried, 3 oz.	34	210	1.0	296	•	.03	.06	2.7	2
Heart, beef, lean, braised, 3 oz.	5	154	5.0	197	20	.21	1.04	6.5	1

Food	Calcium (mg)	Phosphorus (mg)	Iron (mg)	Potassium (mg)	Vitamin A (I.U.)	Thiamin (mg)	Riboflavin (mg)	Niacin (mg)	Ascorbic acid (mg)
Honey, strained or extracted, 1 tbsp.	1	1	.1	11	0	T	.01	.1	T
Honeydew (with rind and seed cavity, 6½ in. diam., 5¼ lb.), 1/10 melon with rind	21	24	.6	374	60	.06	.04	.9	34
Ice Cream:									
Regular (about 11% fat): Hardened, 1 cup	176	134	.1	257	540	.05	.33	.1	1
Soft serve (frozen custard), 1 cup	236	199	.4	338	790	.08	.45	.2	1
Rich (about 16% fat), hardened, 1 cup	151	115	.1	221	900	.04	.28	.1	1
Ice Milk:									
Hardened (about 4.3% fat), 1 cup	176	129	.1	265	210	.08	.35	.1	1
Soft serve (about 2.6% fat), 1 cup	274	202	.3	412	180	.12	.54	.2	1
Jams and preserves, 1 tbsp.	4	2	.2	18	T	T	.01	T	1
Jellies, 1 tbsp.	4	1	.3	14	T	T	.01	T	T
Kale, cooked, drained: From raw (leaves without stems and midribs), 1 cup	206	64	1.8	243	9,130	.11	.20	1.8	102

Foods, approximate measures, units and weight (edible part unless footnotes indicate otherwise)	Grams	Water Percent	Food Energy Calories	Protein Grams	Fat (Total) Grams	Saturated (Total) Grams	Unsaturated Oleic Grams	Linoleic Grams	Carbohydrate Grams
Lamb, cooked:									
Chop, rib (cut 3 per lb. with bone), broiled:									
Lean and fat, 3.1 oz.	8	139	1.0	200	•	.11	.19	4.1	•
Leg, roasted:									
Lean and fat (2 pieces, 4⅛ by 2¼ by ¼ in.), 3 oz.	9	177	1.4	241	•	.13	.23	4.7	•
Shoulder, roasted:									
Lean and fat (3 pieces, 2½ by 2½ by ¼ in.), 3 oz.	9	146	1.0	206	•	.11	.20	4.0	•
Lard, 1 tbsp.	0	0	0	0	10	0	0	0	0
Lemonade concentrate, frozen: Diluted with 4⅓ parts water by volume, 1 cup	2	3	.1	40	50	.01	.02	.2	17
Lemon juice: Raw, 1 cup	17	24	.5	344		.07	.02	.2	112

Food									
Lemon, raw, size 165, without peel and seeds (about 4 per lb. with peels and seeds), 1 lemon	19	12	.4	102	10	.03	.01	.1	39
Lentils, whole, cooked, 1 cup	50	238	4.2	498	40	.14	.12	1.2	0
Lettuce, raw:									
Butterhead, as Boston types:									
Leaves, 1 outer or 2 inner or 3 heart leaves	5	4	.3	40	150	.01	.01	T	1
Crisphead, as Iceberg:									
Pieces, chopped or shredded, 1 cup	11	12	.3	96	180	.03	.03	.2	3
Looseleaf (bunching varieties including romain or cos), chopped or shredded pirces, 1 cup	37	14	.8	145	1,050	.03	.04	.2	10
Limeade concentrate, frozen:									
Diluted with 4⅓ parts water by volume, 1 cup	3	3	T	32	T	T	T	T	6
Lime juice:									
Raw, 1 cup	22	27	.5	256	20	.05	.02	.2	79
Liquor, gin, rum, vodka, whisky:									
80 proof, 1½ fl. oz. jigger	•••	•••	•••	1	•••	•••	•••	•••	•••
86 proof, 1½ fl. oz. jigger	•••	•••	•••	1	•••	•••	•••	•••	•••
90 proof, 1½ fl. oz. jigger	•••	•••	•••	1	•••	•••	•••	•••	•••

Foods, approximate measures, units and weight (edible part unless footnotes indicate otherwise)	Calcium	Phosphorus	Iron	Potassium	Vitamin A Value	Thiamin	Riboflavin	Niacin	Ascorbic Acid
	Milligrams	Milligrams	Milligrams	Milligrams	International units	Milligrams	Milligrams	Milligrams	Milligrams
Liver, beef, fried (slice, 2⅜ by 2⅜ by ⅜ in.), 3 oz.	9	405	7.5	323	45,390	.22	3.56	14.0	23
Macaroni, enriched, cooked (cut lengths, elbows, shells):									
Firm stage (hot), 1 cup	14	85	1.4	103	0	.23	.13	1.8	0
Tender stage:									
Cold macaroni, 1 cup	8	53	.9	64	0	.15	.08	1.2	0
Hot macaroni, 1 cup	11	70	1.3	85	0	.20	.11	1.5	0
Margarine:									
Regular (1 brick or 4 sticks per lb.):									
Tablespoon (about ⅛ stick), 1 tbsp.	3	3	T	4	470	T	T	T	0
Whipped (6 sticks per lb.):									
Tablespoon (about ⅛ stick), 1 tbsp.	2	2	T	2	310	T	T	T	0

	•	•	•	•	•	T	.03	.2	•
Meat, potted (beef, chicken, turkey), canned, 1 tbsp.						T	.03	.2	2
Milk:									
Fluid:									
Whole (3.3% fat), 1 cup	291	228	.1	370	310	.09	.40	.2	2
Lowfat (2%):									
No milk solids added, 1 cup	297	232	.1	377	500	.10	.40	.2	2
Lowfat (1%):									
No milk solids added, 1 cup	300	235	.1	381	500	.10	.41	.2	2
Nonfat (skim):									
No milk solids added, 1 cup	302	247	.1	406	500	.09	.37	.2	2
Buttermilk, 1 cup	285	219	.1	371	80	.08	.38	.1	2
Canned:									
Evaporated, unsweetened:									
Whole milk, 1 cup	657	510	.5	764	610	.12	.80	.5	5
Skim milk, 1 cup	738	497	.7	845	1,000	.11	.79	.4	3
Sweetened, condensed, 1 cup	868	775	.6	1,136	1,000	.28	1.27	.6	8
Dried:									
Buttermilk, 1 cup	1,421	1,119	.4	1,910	260	.47	1.90	1.1	7
Nonfat, instant:									
Cup, 1 cup	837	670	.2	1,160	1,160	.28	1.19	.6	4

Foods, approximate measures, units and weight (edible part unless footnotes indicate otherwise)	Calcium Milli-grams	Phosphorus Milli-grams	Iron Milli-grams	Potassium Milli-grams	Vitamin A Value Internat'l. units	Thiamin Milli-grams	Ribo-flavin Milli-grams	Niacin Milli-grams	Ascorbic Acid Milli-grams
Muffins made with enriched flour:									
From home recipe:									
Blueberry, 2⅜ in. diam., 1½ in. high, 1 muffin	34	53	.6	46	90	.09	.10	.7	T
Bran, 1 muffin	57	162	1.5	172	90	.07	.10	1.7	T
Corn (enriched degermed cornmeal (and flour), 2⅜ in. diam., 1½ in. high, 1 muffin	42	68	.7	54	120	.10	.10	.7	T
Plain, 3 in. diam., 1½ in. high, 1 muffin	42	60	.6	50	40	.09	.12	.9	T
Mushrooms, raw sliced or chopped, 1 cup	4	81	.6	290	T	.07	.32	2.9	2
Mustard, prepared, yellow, 1 tsp. or individual serving pouch or cup	4	4	.1	7	•	•	•	•	•

Mustard greens, without stems and midribs, cooked, drained, 1 cup	193	45	2.5	308	8,120	.11	.20	.8	67
Noodles (egg), enriched, cooked, 1 cup	16	94	1.4	70	110	.22	.13	1.9	0
Oils, salad or cooking:									
Corn, 1 tbsp.	0	0	0	0	—	0	0	0	0
Olive, 1 tbsp.	0	0	0	0	—	0	0	0	0
Peanut, 1 tbsp.	0	0	0	0	—	0	0	0	0
Safflower, 1 tbsp.	0	0	0	0	—	0	0	0	0
Soybean oil, hydrogenated (partially hardened), 1 tbsp.	0	0	0	0	—	0	0	0	0
Sobean-cottonseed oil blend, hydrogenated, 1 tbsp.	0	0	0	0	—	0	0	0	0
Olives, pickled, canned:									
Green, 4 medium or 3 extra large or 2 giant	8	2	.2	7	40	—	—	—	—
Ripe, Mission, 3 small or 2 large	9	1	.1	2	10	T	T	—	—
Onions:									
Mature:									
Raw:									
Chopped, 1 cup	46	61	.9	267	T	.05	.07	.3	17

Foods, approximate measures, units and weight (edible part unless footnotes indicate otherwise)	Calcium Milli-grams	Phosphorus Milli-grams	Iron Milli-grams	Potassium Milli-grams	Vitamin A Value Internat'l. units	Thiamin Milli-grams	Ribo-flavin Milli-grams	Niacin Milli-grams	Ascorbic Acid Milli-grams
Sliced, 1 cup	31	41	.6	181	T	.03	.05	.2	12
Cooked (whole or sliced), drained, 1 cup	50	61	.8	231	T	.06	.06	.4	15
Young green, bulb (⅜ in. diam.) and white portion of top, 6 onions	12	12	.2	69	T	.02	.01	.1	8
Orange and grapefruit juice: Frozen concentrate:									
Diluted with 3 parts water by volume, 1 cup	20	32	.2	439	270	.15	.02	.7	102
Orange juice: Raw, all varieties, 1 cup	27	42	.5	496	500	.22	.07	1.0	124
Canned, unsweetened, 1 cup	25	45	1.0	496	500	.17	.05	.7	100
Frozen concentrate: Diluted with 3 parts water by volume, 1 cup	25	42	.2	503	540	.23	.03	.9	120

Food									
Oranges, all commercial varieties, raw:									
Whole, 2⅝ in. diam., without peel and seeds (about 2½ per lb. with peel and seeds), 1 orange	54	26	.5	263	260	.13	.05	.5	66
Sections without membranes, 1 cup	74	36	.7	360	360	.18	.07	.7	90
Oysters, raw, meat only (13-19 medium Selects), 1 cup	226	343	13.2	290	740	.34	.43	6.0	•
Pancakes, (4 in. diam.):									
Buckwheat, made from mix (with buckwheat and enriched flours) egg and milk added, 1 cake	59	91	.4	66	60	.04	.05	.2	T
Plain:									
Made from mix with enriched flour, egg and milk added, 1 cake	58	70	.3	42	70	.04	.06	.2	T
Parsley, raw, chopped, 1 tbsp.	7	2	.2	25	300	T	.01	T	6
Parsnips, cooked (diced or 2 in. lengths), 1 cup	70	96	.9	587	50	.11	.12	.2	16

291

Foods, approximate measures, units and weight (edible part unless footnotes indicate otherwise)	Calcium Milli-grams	Phosphorus Milli-grams	Iron Milli-grams	Potassium Milli-grams	Vitamin A Value Internat'l. units	Thiamin Milli-grams	Ribo-flavin Milli-grams	Niacin Milli-grams	Ascorbic Acid Milli-grams
Peaches:									
Raw:									
Whole, 2½ in. diam., peeled, pitted (about 4 per lb. with peels and pits), 1 peach	9	19	.5	202	1,330	.02	.05	1.0	7
Sliced, 1 cup	15	32	.9	343	2,260	.03	.09	1.7	12
Peanuts, roasted in oil, salted (whole, halves, chopped), 1 cup	107	577	3.0	971	•	.46	.19	24.8	0
Peanut butter, 1 tbsp.	9	61	.3	100	•	.02	.02	2.4	0
Pears:									
Raw, with skin, cored:									
Bartlett, 2½ in. diam. (about 2½ per lb. with cores and stems), 1 pear	13	18	.5	213	30	.03	.07	.2	7
Bosc, 2½ in. diam. (about 3 per lb. with cores and stems), 1 pear	11	16	.4	83	30	.03	.06	.1	6

Food									
D'Anjou, 3 in. diam. (about 2 per lb. with cores and stems), 1 pear	16	22	.6	260	40	.04	.08	.2	8
Peas, green:									
Frozen, cooked, drained, 1 cup	30	138	3.0	216	960	.43	.14	2.7	21
Peas, split, dry, cooked, 1 cup	22	178	3.4	592	80	.30	.18	1.8	•
Pecans, chopped or pieces (about 120 large halves), 1 cup	86	341	2.8	712	150	1.01	.15	1.1	2
Pepper, hot, red, without seeds, dried (Ground chili powder, added seasonings), 1 tsp.	5	4	.3	20	1,300	T	.02	.2	T
Peppers, sweet (about 5 per lb. whole), stems and seeds removed:									
Raw, 1 pod	7	16	.5	157	310	.06	.06	.4	94
Cooked, boiled, drained, 1 pod	7	12	.4	109	310	.05	.05	.4	70
Pickles, cucumber:									
Dill, medium, whole, 3¾ in. long, 1¼ in. diam., 1 pickle	17	14	.7	130	70	T	.01	T	4
Fresh-pack, slices 1½ in. diam., ¼ in. thick, 2 slices	5	4	.3	•	20	T	T	T	1

293

Foods, approximate measures, units and weight (edible part unless footnotes indicate otherwise)	Calcium Milli-grams	Phosphorus Milli-grams	Iron Milli-grams	Potassium Milli-grams	Vitamin A Value Internat'l. units	Thiamin Milli-grams	Ribo-flavin Milli-grams	Niacin Milli-grams	Ascorbic Acid Milli-grams
Sweet, gherkin, small, whole, about 2½ in. long, ¾ in. diam., 1 pickle	2	2	.2	•	10	T	T	T	1
Pineapple:									
Raw, diced, 1 cup	26	12	.8	226	110	.14	.05	.3	26
Pineapple juice, unsweetened, canned, 1 cup	38	23	.8	373	130	.13	.05	.5	80
Pizza (cheese) baked, 4¾ in. sector; ⅛ of 12 in. diam. pie, 1 sector	86	89	1.1	67	230	.16	.18	1.6	4
Plums, without pits:									
Raw, Japanese and hybrid (2⅛ in. diam.; about 6½ per lb. with pits), 1 plum	8	12	.3	112	160	.02	.02	.3	4

Food									
Prune-type (1½ in. diam., about 15 per lb. with pits), 1 plum	3	5	.1	48	80	.01	.01	.1	1
Popcorn, popped:									
Plain, large kernel, 1 cup	1	17	.2	•	•	•	.01	.1	0
With oil (coconut) and salt added, large kernel, 1 cup	1	19	.2	•	•	•	.01	.2	0
Sugar coated, 1 cup	2	47	.5	•	•	•	.02	.4	0
Pork, cured, cooked:									
Ham, light cure, lean and fat, roasted (2 pieces, 4⅛ by 2¼ by ¼ in.), 3 oz.	8	146	2.2	199	0	.40	.15	3.1	•
Luncheon meat:									
Boiled ham, slice (8 per 8 oz. pkg.), 1 oz.	3	47	.8	•	0	.12	.04	.7	•
Canned, spiced or unspiced: Slice, approx. 3 by 2 by ½ in., 1 slice	5	65	1.3	133	0	.19	.13	1.8	•
Chop, loin (cut 3 per lb. with bone), broiled:									
Lean and fat, 2¾ oz.	9	209	2.7	216	0	.75	.22	4.5	•

Foods, approximate measures, units and weight (edible part unless footnotes indicate otherwise)	Calcium	Phosphorus	Iron	Potassium	Vitamin A Value	Thiamin	Ribo-flavin	Niacin	Ascorbic Acid
	Milli-grams	Milli-grams	Milli-grams	Milli-grams	Internat'l. units	Milli-grams	Milli-grams	Milli-grams	Milli-grams
Roast, oven cooked, no liquid added:									
Lean and fat (piece, 2½ by 2½ by ¾ in.), 3 oz.	9	218	2.7	233	0	.78	.22	4.8	•
Shoulder cut, simmered:									
Lean and fat (3 pieces, 2½ by 2½ by ¼ in.), 3 oz.	9	118	2.6	158	0	.46	.21	4.1	•
Pork link (16 per 1 lb. pkg.), cooked, 1 link	1	21	.3	35	0	.10	.04	.5	•
Potato chips, 1¾ by 2½ in oval cross section, 10 chips	8	28	.4	226	T	.04	.01	1.0	3
Potatoes, cooked:									
Baked, peeled after baking (about 2 per lb. raw), 1 potato	14	101	1.1	782	T	.15	.07	2.7	31
Boiled (about 3 per lb. raw): Peeled after boiling, 1 potato	10	72	.8	556	T	.12	.05	2.0	22

Food								
French-fried, strip, 2 to 3½ in. long:								
Prepared from raw, 10 strips	8	56	.7	427	T	.07	.04	1.6	11
Hashed brown, prepared from frozen, 1 cup	28	78	1.9	439	T	.11	.03	1.6	12
Mashed, prepared from—Raw:								
Milk and butter added, 1 cup	50	101	.8	525	360	.17	.11	2.1	19
Potato salad, made with cooked salad dressing, 1 cup	80	160	1.5	798	350	.20	.18	2.8	28
Pretzels, made with enriched flour:								
Thin, twisted, 3¼ by 2¼ by ¼ in., 10 pretzels	13	79	.9	78	0	.20	.15	2.5	0
Prune juice, canned or bottled, 1 cup	36	51	1.8	602	•	.03	.03	1.0	5
Prunes, dried: "softenized," with pits:								
Uncooked, 4 extra large or 5 large prunes	22	34	1.7	298	690	.04	.07	.7	1
Cooked, unsweetened, all sizes, fruit and liquid, 1 cup	51	79	3.8	695	1,590	.07	.15	1.5	2
Puddings:								
From mix (chocolate) and milk:								
Regular (cooked), 1 cup	265	247	.8	354	340	.05	.39	.3	2

Foods, approximate measures, units and weight (edible part unless footnotes indicate otherwise)	Calcium	Phosphorus	Iron	Potassium	Vitamin A Value	Thiamin	Ribo-flavin	Niacin	Ascorbic Acid
	Milli-grams	Milli-grams	Milli-grams	Milli-grams	Internat'l. units	Milli-grams	Milli-grams	Milli-grams	Milli-grams
Instant, 1 cup	374	237	1.3	335	340	.08	.39	.3	2
Pumpkin, canned, 1 cup	61	64	1.0	588	15,680	.07	.12	1.5	12
Radishes, raw (prepackaged) stem ends, rootlets cut off, 4 radishes	5	6	.2	58	T	.01	.01	.1	5
Raisins, seedless:									
Cup, not pressed down, 1 cup	90	146	5.1	1,106	30	.16	.12	.7	1
Raspberries, red:									
Raw, capped, whole, 1 cup	27	27	1.1	207	160	.04	.11	1.1	31
Rhubarb, cooked, added sugar:									
From raw, 1 cup	211	41	1.6	548	220	.05	.14	.8	16
Rice, white, enriched:									
Instant, ready-to-serve, hot, 1 cup	5	31	1.3	•	0	.21	(*)	1.7	0
Long grain:									
Raw, 1 cup	44	174	5.4	170	0	.81	.06	6.5	0
Cooked, served hot, 1 cup	21	57	1.8	57	0	.23	.02	2.1	0

298

Rolls, enriched:

Commercial:

Brown-and-serve (12 per 12 oz. pkg), browned, 1 roll	20	23	.5	25	T	.10	.06	.9	T
Cloverleaf or pan, 2½ in. diam., 2 in. high, 1 roll	21	24	.5	27	T	.11	.07	.9	T
Frankfurter and hamburger (8 per 1½ oz. pkg), 1 roll	30	34	.8	38	T	.16	.10	1.3	T
Hard, 3¾ in. diam., 2 in. high, 1 roll	24	46	1.2	49	T	.20	.12	1.7	T
Hoagie or submarine, 11½ by 3 by 2½ in., 1 roll	58	115	3.0	122	T	.54	.32	4.5	T

Salad dressings:

Commercial:

Blue cheese:

Regular, 1 tbsp.	12	11	T	6	30	T	.02	T	T
Low calorie (5 Cal. per tsp.), 1 tbsp.	10	8	T	5	30	T	.01	T	T

French:

Regular, 1 tbsp.	2	2	.1	13	•	•	•	•	•
Low calorie (5 Cal. per tsp.), 1 tbsp.	2	2	.1	13	•	•	•	•	•

(*) Product may or may not be enriched with riboflavin. Consult the label.

Foods, approximate measures, units and weight (edible part unless footnotes indicate otherwise)	Calcium	Phosphorus	Iron	Potassium	Vitamin A Value	Thiamin	Riboflavin	Niacin	Ascorbic Acid
	Milligrams	Milligrams	Milligrams	Milligrams	Internat'l. units	Milligrams	Milligrams	Milligrams	Milligrams
Italian:									
Regular, 1 tbsp.	2	1	T	2	T	T	T	T	•
Low calorie (2 Cal. per tsp.), 1 tbsp.	T	1	T	2	T	T	T	T	•
Mayonnaise, 1 tbsp.	3	4	.1	5	40	T	.01	T	•
Mayonnaise type:									
Regular, 1 tbsp.	2	4	T	1	30	T	T	T	•
Low calorie (8 Cal. per tsp.), 1 tbsp.	3	4	T	1	40	T	T	T	• T
Tartar sauce, regular, 1 tbsp.	3	4	.1	11	30	T	T	T	T
Thousand Island:									
Regular, 1 tbsp.	2	3	.1	18	50	T	T	T	T
Low calorie (10 Cal. per tsp.), 1 tbsp.	2	3	.1	17	50	T	T	T	T
Salami:									
Dry type, slice (12 per 4 oz. pkg.), 1 slice	1	28	.4	•	•	.04	.03	.5	•

Cooked type, slice (8 per 8 oz. pkg.), 1 slice	3	57	.7	•	•	.07	.07	1.2	•
Salmon, pink, canned, solids and liquid, 3 oz.	167	243	.7	307	60	.03	.16	6.8	•
Sardines, Atlantic, canned in oil, drained solids, 3 oz.	372	424	2.5	502	190	.02	.17	4.6	•
Sauerkraut, canned, solids and liquid, 1 cup	85	42	1.2	329	120	.07	.09	.5	33
Scallops, frozen, breaded, fried, reheated, 6 scallops	•	•	•	•	•	•	•	•	•
Shad, baked with butter or margarine, bacon, 3 oz.	20	266	.5	320	30	.11	.22	7.3	•
Shrimp:									
Canned meat, 3 oz.	98	224	2.6	104	50	.01	.03	1.5	•
French fried, 3 oz.	61	162	1.7	195	•	.03	.07	2.3	•
Soups:									
Canned, condensed:									
Prepared with equal volume of milk:									
Cream of chicken, 1 cup	172	152	.5	260	610	.05	.27	.7	2
Cream of mushroom, 1 cup	191	169	.5	279	250	.05	.34	.7	1
Tomato, 1 cup	168	155	.8	418	1,200	.10	.25	1.3	15

302

Foods, approximate measures, units and weight (edible part unless footnotes indicate otherwise)	Calcium	Phosphorus	Iron	Potassium	Vitamin A Value	Thiamin	Ribo-flavin	Niacin	Ascorbic Acid
	Milli-grams	Milli-grams	Milli-grams	Milli-grams	Internat'l. units	Milli-grams	Milli-grams	Milli-grams	Milli-grams
Prepared with equal volume of water:									
Bean with pork, 1 cup	63	128	2.3	395	650	.13	.08	1.0	3
Beef broth, bouillon, consomme, 1 cup	T	31	.5	130	T	T	.02	1.2	•
Beef noodle, 1 cup	7	48	1.0	77	50	.05	.07	1.0	T
Clam chowder, Manhattan type, (with tomatoes, without milk), 1 cup	34	47	1.0	184	880	.02	.02	1.0	•
Cream of chicken, 1 cup	24	34	.5	79	410	.02	.05	.5	T
Cream of mushroom, 1 cup	41	50	.5	98	70	.02	.12	.7	T
Minestrone, 1 cup	37	59	1.0	314	2,350	.07	.05	1.0	•
Split pea, 1 cup	29	149	1.5	270	440	.25	.15	1.5	1
Tomato, 1 cup	15	34	.7	230	1,000	.05	.05	1.2	12
Vegetable beef, 1 cup	12	49	.7	162	2,700	.05	.05	1.0	•
Vegetarian, 1 cup	20	39	1.0	172	2,940	.05	.05	1.0	•

Food	•	•	•	4	•	•	•	•	•
Dehydrated:									
Bouillon cube, ½ in., 1 cube	42	49	.6	238	30	.05	.03	.3	6
Mixes:									
Unprepared:									
Onion, 1½ oz. pkg.									
Prepared with water:									
Chicken noodle, 1 cup	7	19	.2	19	50	.07	.05	.5	T
Onion, 1 cup	10	12	.2	58	T	T	T	T	2
Tomato vegetable with noodles, 1 cup	7	19	.2	29	480	.05	.02	.5	5
Spaghetti, enriched, cooked:									
Firm stage, "al dente," served hot, 1 cup	14	85	1.4	103	0	.23	.13	1.8	0
Tender stage, served hot, 1 cup	11	70	1.3	85	0	.20	.11	1.5	0
Spaghetti (enriched) in tomato sauce with cheese:									
From home recipe, 1 cup	80	135	2.3	408	1,080	.25	.18	2.3	13
Spaghetti (enriched) with meat balls and tomato sauce:									
From home recipe, 1 cup	124	236	3.7	665	1,590	.25	.30	4.0	22
Spinach:									
Raw, chopped, 1 cup	51	28	1.7	259	4,460	.06	.11	.3	28

303

Foods, approximate measures, units and weight (edible part unless footnotes indicate otherwise)	Calcium	Phosphorus	Iron	Potassium	Vitamin A Value	Thiamin	Riboflavin	Niacin	Ascorbic Acid
	Milligrams	Milligrams	Milligrams	Milligrams	International units	Milligrams	Milligrams	Milligrams	Milligrams
Cooked, drained:									
From raw, 1 cup	167	68	4.0	583	14,580	.13	.25	.9	50
Squash, cooked:									
Summer (all varieties), diced, drained, 1 cup	53	53	.8	296	820	.11	.17	1.7	21
Winter (all varieties), baked, mashed, 1 cup	57	98	1.6	945	8,610	.10	.27	1.4	27
Strawberries:									
Raw, whole berries, capped, 1 cup	31	31	1.5	244	90	.04	.10	.9	88
Frozen, sweetened:									
Sliced, 10 oz. container, 1 container	40	48	2.0	318	90	.06	.17	1.4	151
Whole, 1 lb. container (about 1¾ cups), 1 container	59	73	2.7	472	140	.09	.27	2.3	249
Sunflower seeds, dry, hulled, 1 cup	174	1,214	10.3	1,334	70	2.84	.33	7.8	•

Food									
Sugars:									
Brown, pressed down, 1 cup	187	42	7.5	757	0	.02	.07	.4	0
White:									
Granulated, 1 cup	0	0	.2	6	0	0	0	0	0
Sweet potatoes:									
Cooked (raw, 5 by 2 in.; about 2½ per lb.):									
Baked in skin, peeled, 1 potato	46	66	1.0	342	9,230	.10	.08	.8	25
Candied, 2½ by 2 in. piece, 1 potato	39	45	.9	200	6,620	.06	.04	.4	11
Tangerine, raw, 2⅜ in. diam., size 176, without peel (about 4 per lb. with peels and seeds), 1 tangerine	34	15	.3	108	360	.05	.02	.1	27
Tangerine juice, canned, sweetened, 1 cup	44	35	.5	440	1,040	.15	.05	.2	54
Tomato catsup, 1 tbsp.	3	8	.1	54	210	.01	.01	.2	2
Tomatoes:									
Raw, 2⅗ in. diam. (3 per 12 oz. pkg.), 1 tomato	16	33	.6	300	1,110	.07	.05	.9	28
Tomato juice, canned:									
Cup, 1 cup	17	44	2.2	552	1,940	.12	.07	1.9	39
Tuna, canned in oil, drained solids, 3 oz.	7	199	1.6	•	70	.04	.10	10.1	•

Foods, approximate measures, units and weight (edible part unless footnotes indicate otherwise)	Calcium	Phosphorus	Iron	Potassium	Vitamin A Value	Thiamin	Ribo- flavin	Niacin	Ascorbic Acid
	Milli- grams	Milli- grams	Milli- grams	Milli- grams	Internat'l. units	Milli- grams	Milli- grams	Milli- grams	Milli- grams
Tuna salad, 1 cup	41	291	2.7	•	590	.08	.23	10.3	2
Turkey, roasted, flesh without skin:									
Dark meat, piece, 2½ by 1⅝ by ¼ in., 4 pieces	•	•	2.0	338	•	.03	.20	3.6	•
Light meat, piece, 4 by 2 by ¼ in., 2 pieces	•	•	1.0	349	•	.04	.12	9.4	•
Turnip greens, cooked, drained:									
From raw (leaves and stems), 1 cup	252	49	1.5	•	8,270	.15	.33	.7	68
Turnips, cooked, diced, 1 cup	54	37	.6	291	T	.06	.08	.5	34
Veal, medium fat, cooked, bone removed:									
Cutlet (4⅛ by 2¼ by ½ in.), braised or broiled, 3 oz.	9	196	2.7	258	•	.06	.21	4.6	•
Rib (2 pieces, 4⅛ by 2¼ by ¼ in.), roasted 3 oz.	10	211	2.9	259	•	.11	.26	6.6	•

Vegetables, mixed, frozen, cooked, 1 cup	46	115	2.4	348	9,010	.22	.13	2.0	15
Vienna sausage (7 per 4 oz. can), 1 sausage	1	24	.3	•	••	.01	.02	.4	••
Vinegar, cider, 1 tbsp.	1	1	.1	15	•	•	•	.	
Waffles, made with enriched flour, 7 in. diam.:									
From home recipe, 1 waffle	85	130	1.3	109	250	.17	.23	1.4	T
From mix, egg and milk added, 1 waffle	179	257	1.0	146	170	.14	.22	.9	T
Walnuts:									
Black:									
Chopped or broken kernels, 1 cup	T	713	7.5	575	380	.28	.14	.9	••
Ground (finely), 1 cup	T	456	4.8	368	240	.18	.09	.6	••
Watermelon, raw, 4 by 8 in. wedge with rind and seeds (1/16 of 32⅔ lb. melon, 10 by 16 in.), 1 wedge with rind and seeds	30	43	2.1	426	2,510	.13	.13	.9	30
Wheat flours:									
All-purpose or family flour, enriched:									
Sifted, spooned, 1 cup	18	100	3.3	109	0	.74	.46	6.1	0

Foods, approximate measures, units and weight (edible part unless footnotes indicate otherwise)	Calcium	Phosphorus	Iron	Potassium	Vitamin A Value	Thiamin	Riboflavin	Niacin	Ascorbic Acid
	Milligrams	Milligrams	Milligrams	Milligrams	International units	Milligrams	Milligrams	Milligrams	Milligrams
Unsifted, spooned, 1 cup	20	109	3.6	119	0	.80	.50	6.6	0
Cake or pastry flour, enriched, sifted, spooned, 1 cup	16	70	2.8	91	0	.61	.38	5.1	0
Self-rising, enriched, unsifted, spooned, 1 cup	331	583	3.6	•	0	.80	.50	6.6	0
Whole wheat, from hard wheats, stirred, 1 cup	49	446	4.0	444	0	.66	.14	5.2	0
White sauce, medium, with enriched flour, 1 cup	288	233	.5	348	1,150	.12	.43	.7	2
Wines:									
Dessert, 3½ fl. oz. glass	8	•	•	77	•	.01	.02	.2	•
Table, 3½ fl. oz. glass	9	10	.4	94	•	T	.01	.1	•
Yogurt:									
With added milk solids:									
Made with lowfat milk:									
Fruit flavored, 1 container, net wt. 8 oz.	343	269	.2	439	120	.08	.40	.2	1

Plain, 1 container, net wt. 8 oz.	415	326	.2	531	150	.10	.49	.3	2
Made with nonfat milk, 1 container, net wt. 8 oz.	452	355	.2	579	20	.11	.53	.3	2
Without added milk solids: Made with whole milk, 1 container, net wt. 8 oz.	274	215	.1	351	280	.07	.32	.2	1

SOURCE: Adapted from L. Patrick Coyle, *The World Encyclopedia of Food* (New York: Facts On File, 1982), pp. 432–475.

Index